VIDEO

Arts for Health

Series Editor: Paul Crawford, Professor of Health Humanities, University of Nottingham, UK

The *Arts for Health* series offers a ground-breaking set of books that guide the general public, carers and healthcare providers on how different arts can help people to stay healthy or improve their health and well-being.

Bringing together new information and resources underpinning the health humanities (that link health and social care disciplines with the arts and humanities), the books demonstrate the ways in which the arts offer people worldwide a kind of shadow health service – a non-clinical way to maintain or improve our health and well-being. The books are aimed at general readers along with interested arts practitioners seeking to explore the health benefits of their work, health and social care providers and clinicians wishing to learn about the application of the arts for health, educators in arts, health and social care and organizations, carers and individuals engaged in public health or generating healthier environments. These easy-to-read, engaging short books help readers to understand the evidence about the value of arts for health and offer guidelines, case studies and resources to make use of these non-clinical routes to a better life.

Other titles in the series:

Film	Steven Schlozman
Theatre	Sydney Cheek-O'Donnell
Singing	Yoon Irons and Grenville Hancox
Reading	Philip Davis
Drawing	Curie Scott
Photography	Susan Hogan
Storytelling	Michael Wilson
Music	Eugene Beresin
Painting	Francisco Javier Saavedra-Macías, Samuel Arias-Sánchez, and Ana Rodríguez-Gómez
Magic	Richard Wiseman
Body Art	Brian Brown and Virginia Kuulei Berndt

Forthcoming titles:

VIDEO

JOHN QUIN

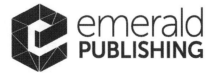

United Kingdom – North America – Japan – India
Malaysia – China

Emerald Publishing Limited
Howard House, Wagon Lane, Bingley BD16 1WA, UK

First edition 2023

British Library Cataloguing in Publication Data
A catalogue record for this book is available from the British Library

ISBN: 978-1-83753-759-4 (Print)
ISBN: 978-1-83753-756-3 (Online)
ISBN: 978-1-83753-758-7 (Epub)

Printed and bound by CPI Group (UK) Ltd, Croydon, CR0 4YY

INVESTOR IN PEOPLE

To Maureen

CONTENTS

ABOUT THE AUTHOR

John Quin is a retired Consultant Physician specializing in general medicine, diabetes and endocrinology. His first book, *Dr. Quin, Medicine Man*, received a four-star review in *The Times*. He has been writing on art, literature and music for more than 20 years for publications including *ArtReview*, *frieze*, *The Quietus*, *Tagesspiegel*, *The Wire*, *The National*, *The Irish Times*, *The Guardian*, *The BMJ* and *The Lancet*.

FOREWORD: CREATIVE PUBLIC HEALTH

The *Arts for Health* series aims to provide key information on how different arts and humanities practices can support, or even transform, health and well-being. Each book introduces a particular creative activity or resource and outlines its place and value in society, the evidence for its use in advancing health and well-being, and cases of how this works. In addition, each book provides useful links and suggestions to readers for following-up on these quick reads. We can think of this series as a kind of shadow health service – encouraging the use of the arts and humanities alongside all the other resources on offer to keep us fit and well.

Creative practices in the arts and humanities offer a fantastic, non-medical, but medically relevant way to improve the health and well-being of individuals, families and communities. Intuitively, we know just how important creative activities are in maintaining or recovering our best possible lives. For example, imagine that we woke up tomorrow to find that all music, books or films had to be destroyed, learn that singing, dancing or theatre had been outlawed or that galleries, museums and theatres had to close permanently; or, indeed, that every street had posters warning citizens of severe punishment for taking photographs, drawing or writing. How would we feel? What would happen to our bodies and minds? How would we survive? Unfortunately, we have seen this kind of removal of creative activities from human society before and today many people remain terribly restricted in artistic expression and consumption.

I hope that this series adds a practical resource to the public. I hope people buy these little books as gifts for family and friends, or for hard-pressed healthcare professionals, to encourage them to revisit or to consider a creative path to living well. I hope that creative public health makes for a brighter future.

Professor Paul Crawford

ACKNOWLEDGEMENTS

I'd like to thank the following people who have encouraged/ mentored/edited my writing over many years: Chris Paling, Martin Herbert, Robert Barry, Luke Turner, John Doran, David Terrien and Mark Rappolt. More recent help has come from Pavithra Muthu and S. Rajachitra of *Emerald Publishing Ltd.*, Laura Webster at *The National* and Martin Doyle of *The Irish Times*. My agent Kevin Pocklington from *The North* continues to bat for me with great persistence at the crease.

I also want to thank the artists who have talked to me for this book: Douglas Gordon, Jacqueline Donachie and Christine Borland. Also to Anri Sala, Oliver Basciano, Nicola Jeffs and Paul Morrish for making suggestions after reading the text.

Extra special thanks to DotMD, the amazing team in Galway: Ronan Kavanagh, Alan Coss and Muiris Houston. Also to Steven Schlozman whose earlier volume in the series – *Film* – proved such a great inspiration.

And to Maureen: yellow blue vase.

The fact that 'normal' people can get around, can see, can hear, doesn't mean that they are seeing or hearing. They can be blind to the things that spoil their happiness, very deaf to the pleas of others for kindness; when I think of them I do not feel any more crippled or disabled than they. Perhaps in some small way I can be the means of opening their eyes to the beauties around us; things like a warm handclasp, a voice that is anxious to cheer, a spring breeze, music to listen to, a friendly nod. These people are important to me, and I like to feel that I can help them.

A patient with multiple sclerosis quoted in 'Stigma' by Erving Goffman.

I would sit right down, waiting for the gift of sound and vision.

David Bowie

INTRODUCTION AND A BRIEF HISTORY: WHY VIDEO? WHY VIDEO ART?

THE SEA, THE SEA

The day after the proposal for this book was accepted I walked, on an odd impulse, to the Fabrica Gallery in Brighton, a converted Regency church that sits nestled among the many coffee shops and restaurants in the city's centre. It was dark under the wooden rafters, but I made my way into a curtained-off section where two large adjoining screens showed a video work by Vanessa Daws, a Dublin-based artist. What I saw projected was the bobbing sea, an endless vista of waves, the waters of what might be a channel or an ocean, who knew? A woman's voice then talked over the images. She spoke about wild swimming and the challenge of long-distance crawls. The artwork was called *At Home in the Water*. The visuals were mesmeric and it was easy to zone out, drift into a Zen-like meditative state, as I watched a swimmer's arms plunging and rising again and again into the choppy white horses. I could imagine coming here after a long shift, a tired healthcare worker in need of balm and calm, then relaxing, relaxing.

But art asks much more of us than a mere *c'mon, chill out*. The art was intended to make the viewer think – what is this work *really* about? Were we meant to consider exercise and the vigorous appeal of extreme effort? To some extent, but this wasn't a fitness-instruction video. There was something else, something more expansive, more ambitious, going on ... and then it hit me.

Daws' video could be seen as a metaphor for video art *itself*: video as opposed to movies. What we were watching was something

1

utterly plot-less and potentially near infinite, and yet extremely easy to dip in and out of. You didn't have to be there right at the start of the film, you didn't need to stick around until the end. *This wasn't a movie!* Video art works could be imagined as the sea, or an ocean, a boundless form that we've not entirely explored as yet, a medium not utterly navigated. Video could be treated as an art form that could easily, as with movies, have relevance to medicine and healthcare, one in which we might immerse ourselves in for minutes – as in a short bath – or hours as in one of Daws' long-distance swims.

And now, in the twenty-first century, we are in a new floating world – as the Japanese might say – of video and video technology. We inhabit a transient, unreliable place – an updated *ukiyo* culture – where we live in the moment online. We are immersed (a word overused in art criticism but entirely appropriate here), some might say drowning, in a permanent now on social media. Many people have even given up on television as such; the physical sets being too bulky, too uncool, too immobile for our near-permanent ambulatory lives. We now watch clips on Instagram, YouTube, TikTok, Twitter: choose your platform. We submerge in and out of our tablets and mobile phones on the train, on the bus, in search of entertainment and enlightenment.

Healthcare is no exception to this new paradigm. Got a query on a ward round? No more of those educational prescriptions that involved a trip to the library to consult actual *physical* books: just open up Google and ask away. The answer is in your pocket. The implications of this new technology for medical teaching are enormous and not yet fully understood; already the role of the traditional lecture is being seriously questioned. Students might fall asleep after 10 minutes unless you've got the stand-up skills of a top comedian (Bradbury, 2016).

Open Twitter and you'll see quizzes on X-rays, ECG interpretation, spot diagnoses; immediate learning that sits benignly between scrolling over news headlines like a brief portal into *actual* wisdom. This book is thus based on the proposal that both video art and videos available on social media platforms may be helpful in educating both healthcare workers *and* patients alike. As far as I'm aware this idea has not, as yet, been formally tested scientifically to any great extent, but my hope is that this book will make a strong argument for its further study.

As a corollary, many of my proposals/suggestions here are necessarily speculative. The need for research has become particularly urgent given the immense and growing popularity of social media. These outlets often highlight video works, often short and to the point. Some have a high likelihood of impacting on health behaviours. Most cannot be considered as artworks as such but many are clearly un-ignorable.

While the bulk of this book will address video as an art form the recent mutation of video usage into social media outlets will also be examined and we will highlight specific healthcare related examples. To continue the earlier oceanic metaphor about video this selection will be as random as dipping a fishing net into the deep. There are millions of personal statements from patients out there; many appear helpful, some less so. I've trawled a haul and selected ones that strike me as being particularly powerful. This then is a particularly personal sample. Readers will find their own particular favourites out there.

I've also picked a small number of significant episodes from TV history for discussion but I have deliberately decided to avoid the large number of medical TV dramas, these being (arguably) the subject for entirely different volume. Video is a protean medium and there's the sense that we are still in the foothills of its evolution.

VIDEO VS CINEMA

We should try to make an early distinction between cinematic film and video despite clear overlaps. This differentiation is not clear-cut. Steven Schlozman has addressed film in an earlier volume in this series. He deals with the role cinematic works might play in influencing healthcare and its potential use for patients. The same principle applies here in *Video* although, as said, there is not nearly as much scientific study as regards the impact of video art in comparison to cinema. One has the strong suspicion that many of the conclusions of the scientific studies on movies highlighted in Schlozman's volume could equally apply to video art. *Video* will deal with visual art works and short clips on social media that are *not* mainstream movie productions. *Video* will not concern itself with less commercial art house films that still involve standard cinematic tropes like plot, acting skills and so on.

The key advantage of video over film, as far as its impact as an art form is concerned, an art form that may help healthcare workers and patients understand their world, is *time*. It takes time to head out to a movie, or watch one at home. You need to invest a significant amount of attention to pick up on plot and its exposition. You need to identify with characters. We all love movies, as Schlozman brilliantly demonstrates, but sometimes we just don't have the time to see one. Video works can fill that gap. Video works can give you a message that's instant.

There's a famous scene in Nic Roeg's movie *The Man Who Fell to Earth* (1976) where David Bowie, playing an alien, screams 'Get out of my mind!' to a bank of TV sets blaring multiple voices, multiple sets of imagery. This overabundance of video could be feared; many have worried about potential deleterious effects on mental health. But Roeg was probably being too pessimistic about our capacities to take in screeds of information. The brain is much cleverer than we know. Nowadays most of us take this profusion of messaging as the norm ....

Video art works are of course generally aimed at an art-gallery-going audience, not mainstream cinemagoers. Some video artists have progressed onto longer film works but these are only rarely, if ever, shown in standard cinemas. Even rarer still are those video artists who have evolved into full-on movie directors. But I'd want to stress that gallery going is *not* absolutely essential for the appreciation of video art: it remains the best way *aesthetically* to appreciate the work but for educational purposes much is now available online. A quick survey of the many works mentioned in this book would take about the same time to watch as a single Hollywood production.

This volume will also consider a few exemplary TV moments that are easily available on YouTube. Of course, *Video* could never be an utterly comprehensive survey. The selection of artists here is invariably linked to personal taste. I'm reminded, to continue that earlier aquatic metaphor, of writer Adam Nicolson's (2021) thoughts on the coast and how 'the closer you look, the deeper it dives'. Video as form might be compared to the famed Mandelbrot set, it's a world of fractals: one video leads on inexorably to another like the convolutions of a coastline. Witness the popularity of Instagram and TikTok feeds where you can scroll clips for hours on end. Commercial algorithms exploit this rapacity; this fact in itself might argue for the select group of suggestions that *Video* proposes.

Video will thus examine several clinically relevant aspects of medical practice that have been the topic of video art works. As said, there is no intention here to be comprehensive as this would be an impossible task: the sheer volume of material out there on the Internet is enormous. And the rapidity and ease of access is stunning. Works that previously could only be accessed by a gallery visit are now easily available online.

Praising cinema's ease of access Schlozman compares it with other art forms and asks in his own introduction: 'How often can you recall or even access an interview with a famous artist whose work you enjoyed at a local gallery?' True – this is not easy to do in real life. But this situation has radically changed with the Internet and YouTube: now you *can* access many such interviews online. Some are cited in *Video*; many are extremely enjoyable and informative. There's now a large library of these, many of which are mentioned in the reference section.

Suggestions will be made in *Video* as to how these works might be used as teaching materials and/or may be useful to discuss with patients and carers dealing with issues varying from new life to bereavement. Appropriately *Video* will start its review with matters relating to birth and death. But first, we need recap the basic history of the medium ....

VIDEO: A SHORT HISTORY

Let's begin with a short outline of developments in video and its use as an art form as distinct from cinema. New York City was the centre of the art world in the 1960s and it was from there that video art came to prominence (London, 2020). Museums were initially somewhat sceptical of the new developments, in particular curators were quite concerned about sound bleeding into silent spaces elsewhere; this was quickly addressed. By common consent, the first major artist to popularize the use of video technology was Nam June Paik (1932–2006). Early video art used *actual* TV sets and today these works can look somewhat clunky in art galleries with their use of outmoded models, grainy imagery and poor sound. This was often, as in Paik's case, art about TV *itself*, and thus of limited relevance to healthcare workers. He used television sets sculpturally; this was art about technology. Many of these works from the 1960s also had serious political intent – the Vietnam War was at its height – and as with Instagram and Twitter use today artists saw an opportunity to get their message across with some urgency. The American artist Carolee Schneeman is thought to have made one of the first anti-war videos.

Famously, the Canadian media theorist Marshall McLuhan said of TV that 'the medium is the message'. By this, he meant, in part, that it was video *itself* that needed to be studied as a form of media, as a form of communication, with particular regard as to the implications of its power. By extension, McLuhan's thinking can be applied today towards social media platforms and their use of video. We need to consider the impact these new forms of media will have on medicine, their effects on patients and on medical education. *Video* will try to provoke such discussion.

Cost of video technology, portable cameras and videotape, was prohibitive to most artists in the 1960s, especially in developing countries, and so it's not surprising that their use was super-specialized. As the price of equipment fell portable video recorders and cassettes (arriving around 1971) became more widely available. Nam June Paik echoed the individualist sentiments of Joseph Beuys when he said 'like pen and paper and canvas … the camera makes everyone an artist'. He was right. Paik was absolutely ahead of the game. Today making a short video clip on your mobile phone is an everyday event for billions.

The new technology had an obvious advantage over film – videotape did not need developing and it was easy to re-record. Artists were attracted by the ease of distribution: all you needed was a TV and a VCR rather than the un-wieldy and costly business of moving sculptures and large paintings around the world. After initial hesitation, museums soon began collecting video works and individuals began collecting too. There are even trained *conservators* of video works today. And the technology just gets better and better: digital imagery is now much more polished. There are serious overlaps with video game technology: young people – healthcare students and patients alike – are highly adept at the use of new modes of communication. As a result, older methods of education are being questioned: we ask – can the message be put across more effectively, more efficiently, with the new tools? McLuhan's mantra remains relevant – we need to interrogate the medium, make it work for us, dismiss what is useless.

Are any of these early works still insightful from a healthcare perspective? Not many. David Hall's *60 TV Sets* (1972) is exactly that, a multiscreen installation that would be later referenced in the said Roeg/Bowie film *The Man Who Fell to Earth*. The work captures the chaotic and incessant flow of information that is now normative in our own time of scrolling and rapid-fire imagery. But it wouldn't be long before video artists addressed the body and health.

VIDEO AND THE BODY

The body quickly became the focus of much video art in the 1970s. Early works by Bruce Nauman and Dan Graham often focussed on the body in space and had implications for neurological studies that we will discuss later. They used mirrors and time-delays to discombobulate the viewer interacting with a camera. More disorientation is seen in Gilbert and George's *Gordon's Makes Us Drunk* (1972) – an amusing study of behaviour during inebriation, instantly recognizable to anyone who works in an A+E environment.

Martha Rosler focussed her attention on women's bodies – with her *Semiotics of the Kitchen* (1975). This is arguably required viewing for women involved in healthcare who *still* face the continued condescension of many male patients and staff: the expectation that a female health worker should behave like a maid, or the regular trial female doctors face when they are addressed as 'nurse', and so on.

Chris Burden's early video works documented several actions that dealt with self-harm; these raise even more complex issues with the body. His work will be discussed at length too in Chapter 3. One issue he highlights relevant to today's world is this: should videos showing self-harm be available on modern media platforms? Issues of freedom of expression come up against the real possibility of harmful influence – as was evident in the UK in the recent past with the case of a young boy who accidently killed himself following a TikTok 'challenge'. There are now even several online lists of dangerous TikTok trends (one has 3.8 million views at last check) and how they can impact children's safety. These may have a useful public health purpose.

ANDY WARHOL

The foundational 1960s influence of Andy Warhol must be referenced. His early time-based works, for example, *Sleep* (1964) are arguably of interest to sleep physicians! These are technically films … but they are clearly *not* serious commercial propositions. Warhol's influence cannot be minimized – his much-quoted maxim 'in the future everyone will be famous for 15 minutes' was mutated by the Scottish musician and artist Momus (Nick Currie) who accurately predicted that in the future everyone would be famous for 15 people. This has come about largely as a result of the explosion in video technology and social platforms. Patients have taken full advantage of such technology, particularly those with rare conditions who can now communicate with others around the globe as a community. There can be distinct advantages to being famous for 15 people if you and the other 15 have the same rare medical problem. The potential use of such self-made videos in medical education will be discussed later.

1970s/1980s

By the 1970s, a newer generation of video artists were making works that were becoming ever more ambitious and strained at the boundaries of the new technology. Scale was one factor that changed significantly as with Bill Viola's works that highlight the body and issues of life and death. These will be addressed in the next chapter.

My own introduction to contemporary art (that I later came to understand as life-changing) was in 1980. The monumental eight-part TV series 'The Shock of the New', written and presented by Robert Hughes, taught me that medicine had much to learn from modern artists. Their own powers of observation and societal diagnosis were to be admired and emulated. Hughes' passion in argument, his pithy erudition, his occasional Antipodean irreverence, made him seem to me as if he were another clinical teacher, another giant who could sharpen my apprenticeship.

By the 1980/1990s, pop video culture was omnipresent; the rise of MTV drove artists to ever-more experimental highs. The interaction with healthcare was not the prime driver at this point – money and pop music were – but still there was the occasional work that dared to deal with illness. Tony Oursler worked with the band Sonic Youth; both were fascinated by the tragic figure of singer Karen Carpenter. They made a video together called *Tunic (Song for Karen)* (1990) that specifically addressed Carpenter's anorexia nervosa. Depending on your point of view this work was either an insightful understanding into American excess or an example of cynical exploitation. What sufferers of anorexia made of it seems unrecorded. Oursler would go on to work with ever-smaller LCD projectors and use these to project images of adult faces onto children's dolls. These had a predictably *umheimlich* effect, a queasy, spooky take on psychological illness and mental ill health issues such as dissociative identity disorder. In time he'd go on to work with David Bowie on the affecting *Where Are We Now* video. Bowie, as with Nam June Paik, was always streets ahead ....

TECHNO-FEAR AND THE NEW LUDDITES

Video technologies have their pessimists like the Peruvian novelist Mario Vargas Llosa who, writing in *Notes on the Death of Culture: Essays on Spectacle and Society*, worries that new technologies favour 'minimal intellectual effort at the expense of commitment, concern and, in the final instance, even of thought itself'. I would suggest that his fears are greatly exaggerated. Our time may have 'given itself over, in a passive manner' to what Marshall McLuhan calls the 'image bath', what Vargas Llosa himself admits can be a 'very brilliant bombardment of images that capture our attention'. But my argument here is that Llosa's concern that these images 'dull our sensibilities and intelligence due to their primary and transitory nature' are ill-founded and mirror similar historical concerns as noted when cinema and TV were first invented.

Likewise, although the cultural theorist Jean Baudrillard's fears of an attack on 'the principle of reality' may have some applicability in the *political* arena – the idea that the communications revolution has, in Llosa's words 'abolished the human ability to tell the difference between truth and lies' is somewhat exaggerated. We need to affirm that propaganda using new technologies is nothing new (we recall the pernicious use of radio by Joseph Goebbels) and that these very advances can have equally powerful positive usages, as with medical education.

A key argument in this book promoting video chimes with Schlozman's conclusions on cinema: video artworks are often about empathy, about sympathy for others. These works try to help us break out of the jail of our own consciousness and inhabit that of the other. We're reminded of Vladimir Nabokov's (1956) fondness for a story about a chimp that could draw and its first image: the bars of its cage. Video helps us escape this solipsistic state.

Video art is less about escapism than the movies. And video art is less 'feel-good' than the movies: its role may even be more 'feel-bad' (!) but in an *instructive* way, it begs us to think again, to question our certainties. We can use the Internet and its access to video as selectively as a skilled sailor circumnavigating those fractal twists of the coastline. We're not chimps, we're not that dumb.

1

BIRTH AND DEATH

BILL VIOLA

Does medicine get any more profound than our daily dealings with birth and death? But it's what we do as healthcare workers; it's our bread and butter. We move like little yachts bobbing through the immense sea of obstetrics and pathology. 'We're all water' as Yoko Ono (more on whom later) says in one of her songs. I'm reminded yet again of Vanessa Daws and her metaphorical video work on swimming. And I'm reminded too of Bill Viola's innovative *Nantes Triptych* (1992). Viola often works with water. He's said that video itself is 'electronic water: (with) its flowing, it flows in circuits'. As a medical registrar, one of my colleagues did research into the flow of blood through arteries and she taught me its term: 'rheology'. We might see video *and* the body as rheological forms, rheological mediums.

Viola takes on the big themes of life: how we got here, how we leave. As with Nabokov's oft-quoted line from *Speak, Memory* we're reminded that 'the cradle rocks above an abyss', the abyss being our non-existence before birth and after death. Viola's use of the triptych form recalls traditional Western religious painting: his quoting of this structuring is quite deliberate with its use of altarpieces and the twin side panels. *Nantes Triptych* covers the body's journey through life and features (on the left-hand screen) a woman in childbirth, while on the right, the artist's mother lies dying in a hospital bed. The middle screen has a single male figure – a self-portrait of Viola immersed in water, himself suspended between birth and death, twisting in the vortex of mid-life. Sound is important; we hear crying, water noises and breathing: all in a 30-minute loop.

Obstetricians and midwives will hone in on the left-hand screen and watch the woman giving birth, the everyday miracle of delivery. A gloved hand aids the process, wipes the baby's head as it appears. With a final yell, the body slips out in a second, and the midwife immediately hands the newborn up to the new mother. 'There's your baby.'

We might also compare Viola's 1990s work to the obstetric phenomenon known as 'the quickening' – the first moments when a pregnant woman can feel foetal movement. *Nantes Triptych* can be thought of as another type of quickening – it is one of the first videos of an actual delivery in process to be viewed by a global audience. Search 'birth' on TikTok now, and you'll find innumerable *actual* scenes of childbirth. To my non-obstetric eyes, this would appear to be a major teaching material resource for midwives and obstetricians as well as being of huge potential use to prospective parents. The clips show you what's going to happen ... some will be reassured, others frightened. But there's no doubting the reality of the clips; these are not staged, or acted or faked. Declining birth rates in developed countries meant that previously many people had no, or little, idea of what the birth process entailed: video has changed all that.

As we watch the delivery in *Nantes Triptych*, we simultaneously see Viola, the central clothed male figure, as he writhes underwater. At the same time, the figure on the right, the old woman, gasps her last. This is the screen I imagine palliative care teams and pathologists will focus on. She dies what can only be described as 'a good death', a peaceful, meaningful death. Viola would make another work on his mum's demise called *The Passing* (1991), where his camera slowly pans over his mother's face and her inutile breathing tube.

As Viola says in a video interview available on YouTube: 'These are the great universal experiences, the most private, personal experiences'. The camera invades privacy – hence, for Viola, an inherent tension. This is a moment that asks: 'Should we be watching this?' And yet, for healthcare workers, what we see in his videos are daily experiences. His work reminds us that, for others, such events are as personal as life (and death) get. Viola's videos have quite obvious relevance and impact for those involved in healthcare. Patients and carers will undoubtedly register the powerful emotional charge of *Nantes Triptych*.

For Viola, video is a means, as with American-Indian notion of the camera, of capturing the soul. Videos are – in his words – 'keepers of the soul, they hold souls' and as such, given technological developments in preservation, and may, potentially, give glimpses into our 'souls' for as long as man exists. Video, as a medium, can hold lives. This idea, that the dead may be kept alive in some way, brings us to the great French artist Christian Boltanski.

CHRISTIAN BOLTANSKI

Boltanski (1944–2021) took death as his subject (Semin, Garb, & Kupsit, 1997). One way of understanding his work is to grasp his horror, our horror, that we are all, eventually, forgotten. Boltanski wants us to be remembered: *all of us*. Hence his appropriation of photographs from obituary notices, photographs of the dead. These he often enlarged, framed and then lit with what can be understood as a votive light bulb. Boltanski was Jewish – his work references the Holocaust – but for Boltanski there's another ongoing Holocaust, the natural form of death that will get us all in time. As for memorializing, he made no distinction between the good and the bad. Some of the nice gentle-looking faces we stare at, now long dead, may have been Nazis. Faces don't give everything away. Faces can be masks.

Boltanski could appear clown-like in some of his works, but he was a very serious artist. As the son of a Jewish physician Boltanski knew that, in his own melancholic words: 'The boss of the café where I have my morning coffee is a nice man. I like him very much, he's a sweet person, but he might kill me'.

Much of Boltanski's work is installational in nature but can be easily viewed online. A key piece is *Reserve: The Dead Swiss* (1989) where we see several rows of monochrome obituary shots of the recently deceased taken from local newspapers. Why the Swiss? Boltanski again:

> *I chose the Swiss because they have no history. It would be awful and disgusting to make a piece using dead Jews – or dead Germans for that matter. But the Swiss have no reason to die, so they could be anyone and everyone, which is why they are universal.*

There's dark humour here of course; he's well aware the Swiss could be considered boring. We recall Orson Welles in *The Third Man* with his line about the kitschy Swiss and their invention of the cuckoo clock. But there's another side to the Swiss; they can be accused of being quietly complicit and profiteering from the Holocaust. Boltanski was not always consistent (who cares? who is?) and in time he would make work about the murdered Jews. The moving photographs featured in *Jewish School of Gross Hamburgerstrasse in Berlin, 1938* (1994) have, like Viola's work, a stunningly emotional import.

And, as with Viola, Boltanski was also acutely aware of his own imminent demise. *The Man Who Coughs* (1969) is precisely that, a short video of a man coughing his guts up. Anyone working on a chest ward will recognize this person, someone with bronchial cancer, someone threatened by an immediate and fatal haemoptysis. And then we see it happen: gouts flow. Is this for real or is it a set-up? Is Boltanski clowning around again? What are we supposed to make of this coughing man? He's a sufferer; he's dying. Boltanski wants us to pity him. But he wants us to be disturbed too. He wants us to face up to the reality of dying. Medical students might do well to see this video before being exposed to the trauma of viewing sudden death from haemoptysis or haematemesis in real life on the wards.

An excerpt from Boltanski's *Subliminal/Les Disparus* (2020) can be viewed on Vimeo. In the gallery setting, this is a four-channel video where images are projected onto large white sheets. What we see is a forest; it appears to be snowing. In another scene, we see some deer in a green field. There's a clichéd sunset and a flock of birds: bucolic images then, obvious visual signifiers for calm and relaxation. But there's dirt behind the daydream (as the Gang of Four pop group would have it). Microseconds of black and white footage are spliced in between these idyllic moments. We briefly recognize shots from the Vietnam War, photographs of bunks in death camps. What we get is long periods of heaven with transient glimpses of hell. Death, for Boltanski, is always lurking, always threatening – as with a superficially calm ward full of mortally sick patients.

STEVE MCQUEEN

McQueen is interested in death too. He's that rare phenomenon: an artist who began his career making video art but who now also makes highly successful movies and TV dramas. He's been acclaimed for productions like *Hunger* (2008), *Shame* (2011), *12 Years a Slave* (2013) and *Small Axe* (2020). As such his work can be used as an exemplar of the differences in style and tone that distinguish video works from more commercial projects. He's brilliantly talented at both storytelling – as per his movies – skilled at giving us an arc of a tale that begins and ends with concision. But he also gives us the circular, endlessly repeated imagery of his video artworks. *Five Easy Pieces* (1995) is a good example of the latter as we follow a woman who crosses a tightrope. The camera is underneath her feet as she takes the tentative steps. McQueen himself thinks this 'the perfect image of a combination of vulnerability and strength'. Anyone who has had to perform a difficult technical procedure in medicine – emergency cardiac pacing for example – will understand this work.

The video of McQueen's that has the most relevance to our focus here on life and death and medical care is *Ashes* (2002–2015). This is a 20-minute loop of film. Made with footage taken over ten years on the island of Grenada, we see a young man in the prime of life sitting on a boat in the Caribbean; the blues of the sea and sky are entirely seductive. The man has dyed blonde dreadlocks. His nickname is the sadly ironic title of the work – 'Ashes'. He beams at us: you think – *can anyone look more alive?* Projected on the other side of the screen is the other side of life, or rather death,

Ashes' death. We hear his story told by locals – how Ashes discovered a cache of drugs, how he stole them, how he met his death. He was murdered by drug dealers and then buried in an unmarked grave. What we then see on the other side of the screen is his re-burial. We watch his headstone being carved, hear the bang of hammers and saws grinding away. We see the etching of an inscription. We see the dust that results from the incised marble. We pick up the echo with his name; Ashes was only 25 years when he died. We see a lot of work goes into making a grave. As Celina Colby (2017) writes of the loop, the circle of life here: 'We see Ashes and the gravediggers whose labour is how they make their bread and butter'. As Colby notes: 'His death is their life'.

The contrast between the two sides of the screen – the magnificence of life on the one, the dreadful loss of death on the other – is simply achieved but the impact is direct and to the heart: *What a waste of a life.* What a waste of the beauty of life; Ashes was shot in the back. As McQueen himself has said 'life and death have always been side by side in all aspects of life. Our day-to-day life is full of ghosts'.

ED ATKINS/STAN BRAKHAGE

The Act of Seeing With One's Own Eyes was a project curated by the British artist Ed Atkins in Berlin. The title referred to a notorious 1971 film by Stan Brakhage (1933–2003). A notice in the exhibition warned about explicit contents before you pushed at the smoked glass doors to see the work inside. Let's go in ….

Brakhage was a highly regarded experimental filmmaker, the creator of abstract imagery featuring blotches and scratches on celluloid that one might associate with an accompaniment of psychedelic music. The grainy 16mm film shown by Atkins in Berlin was *very* different. What we see is a group of Pittsburgh pathologists at work in a mortuary. The film is also silent; it lasts an intense 32 minutes. Cadavers are seen on gurneys, some covered in white sheets, others lie prone on steel tables. There is much blood, and there are brains cupped in the living hands of the pathologists as they slip out from open skulls. Sad dead feet flop about unintentionally as the body is manipulated more cranially, out of shot. The film is *not* a pedagogic work for medical students. Brakhage's footage is art in the same sense that Rembrandt's painting *The Anatomy Lesson of Dr. Nicolaes Tulp* (1632) was art; these works make us think about that frail thing we all are: a body.

Watching the various corpses being dissected – the heads being incised, the voids of the abdominal cavities exposed and then flushed out, the organs weighed and measured – all this gives rise to many questions about the nature of observation. We might break these enquiries down and observe the reactions of four interested parties: firstly – and predominant – there is our own response; secondly there is that of our peers here – the other members of the audience; thirdly there's that of filmmaker Brakhage himself, and finally the intentions of Atkins as curator.

A caveat: I've been here before, for real, having attended many post-mortems. The medical gaze (that of doctors and pathologists) is predominantly that of the distanced scientist who asks coldly: *what has happened to this person?* What is/are the cause(s) of death? For a medic, there is a degree of frustration watching Brakhage's film in the sense that we want to know more about the aetiology of the individual's demise. We see a thumb imprint itself in the oedema of an ankle and assume cardiac or liver or kidney failure as being a contributory cause of death. There are what appear to be dialysis lines in another cadaver. Other bodies have injuries that intrigue with the possibility of murder, assault and criminal involvement. But Brakhage deliberately excludes us from making swift and facile conclusions with his sharp and fast editing, his own fearless cutting. This film cannot be explicated with ease.

Some visitors will fear the imagery of dissection. Many doctors are just as scared of pathologists as the general public. They dread the phone call that asks that they come down to the morgue where they will be confronted with the stark reality of a misdiagnosis, the incorrect interpretation of an X-ray, the operation gone wrong.

As said the film is silent – it's a true *stummfilm* – and the lack of sound (when I attended a showing) was if anything intensified by the stunned audience. Scanning the pallid faces as people left the room I saw horrified Japanese women lifting hands to their faces,

German hipsters affecting a phony *sangfroid* – a contrived 'seen it all before' pose, some black-suited academics trying to preserve their cool. There was an air of bravado from some of the others, as with school kids on a visit to an anatomy museum. A few were deliberately here to see the transgressive – *shock me!* They were here to stare at what they have never seen before, to look at Brakhage's imagery with a prurient, voyeuristic intent, as if glimpsing pornography for the first time.

And indeed Brakhage does not spare us. The handling of the bodies appears rough, insensitive. We see a huge syringe draining what might be an effusion on a lung, other internal cavities being sluiced like carcases at an abattoir. Reproductive organs are exposed brutally, muted of all erotic association. This is what being dead looks like and it's for real.

What of Brakhage's intentions? He is interested in the day-to-day business of how pathologists work – this is what he shows us here, how our beloved bodies are reduced to a mere object for study. And what about the aims of Atkins as curator? I'll have more to say about his work in Chapter 8 but here he's interested in how we wilfully try to tame the unbearable, the horrific final state of our form, the true fate of the body. A line from John le Carré's *Smiley's People* (1979) chimes with Atkins' thinking on Brakhage's work. Lacon, a politician, is sympathizing with spymaster George Smiley who has just witnessed a corpse with its face blown off:

'Was it gruesome, George? How perfectly awful for you.'

No, it wasn't awful, it was the truth, thought Smiley.

TV 1: MY DEAD BODY

Here's Claire Smith, the Professor of Anatomy based at my own hospital and medical school in Brighton. She's talking about 'an extra special donor', a young woman – Toni Crews – who died aged only 30 years with a rare form of cancer affecting one of her tear glands. Toni gave the department special consent to use her body for anatomical examination and public display. This in turn meant that the anatomists could, along with consent from the family, 'trace the journey of cancer and teach a wide range of students'. There were 12 workshops teaching over 800 students. As part of the process, the team worked with a TV production company to make a video documentary.

Unsurprisingly, the TV programme had a significant impact and was well reviewed. Lucy Mangan (2022) in *The Guardian* noted 'the truth of it (the autopsy) is not shied away from' but also praises the filmmakers' 'commendable restraint'. The bulk of the documentary is about Toni's life that includes some of her own social media posts and home videos – another example of how video and its ability to capture self-portraiture can be hugely informative and helpful in medical education. As Mangan concludes: 'You don't have to be in the lecture hall with Smith and her students to feel you have been enlarged and educated by Toni's presence'.

TV 2: DENNIS POTTER

Television – although primarily seen as pure entertainment rather than art – can, occasionally, provide healthcare workers with pure gold. Again there is ease of access as with the many TV plays available on DVD or the large number of clips from TV interviews about healthcare existing on YouTube. Let's talk about one of the most famous.

An empty TV studio, two seats with side tables for drinks. Figures walk in from the darkness: two men in suit and tie, formal. 'Mine's with the ashtray' says a bespectacled figure gesturing at the seats. This is the playwright Dennis Potter and this is his last televised interview; the other man is the novelist and presenter, Melvyn Bragg. What follows is extraordinary, what follows should be mandatory viewing for those involved in palliative care and for all of us staring at death. As they settle into their seats there's a brief discussion about a silver hipflask. Potter, now seated, says: 'I'll only need it if there's any spasms'. An assistant adds: 'Melvyn can pass it to you …'.

Potter is 59 years and he's dying from pancreatic cancer; he has liver metastases and the hipflask contains liquid opiate. He says he's still driving himself – 'I've got to keep moving with the pain so

I've got my pen in my hand'. Lesson one then about the dying – not all turn to the wall. For some, it's the great stimulant to work. He has a glass of white wine in one hand, a ciggie in the other; he's clearly in pain. The frown lines are deep but he remains fluent, taking care with each and every word as if it were his last. He has a schedule of work and starts at 5.00 a.m. He makes jokes about attending to his affairs.

He admits to worrying about being a coward but says he cares more about his family and friends than himself. He focusses on the present tense, what the singer Momus calls 'the nowness of now'. Potter celebrates the trivial and the important, the glory of blossom outside his house: 'if you see the present tense ... boy, can you see it, boy can you celebrate it'.

Bragg's interviewing style and his questioning beg to be studied by all involved in breaking bad news, in counselling the dying. Bragg is a great listener and gives Potter all the space he needs for his eloquent thoughts. He's after Potter's wisdom and knows that the man he's interviewing can teach us all given his insights into life, childhood, love and loss. Bragg's questions are open and he laughs with Potter at appropriate moments; this is not a wake. Potter is still very much alive as he grasps at his lighter, as he fires up another cigarette. It's way too late for disapproval, too late for medical tut-tutting.

Look closer at Potter's hands: there's the skewed malformations, the sausage-like fingers and swellings of psoriatic arthropathy. Potter gave his own condition to one of his greatest characters – *The Singing Detective*. At one point he raises his crippled limbs to Bragg and, with black humour, talks of his psoriasis itching away: 'Which is a bugger, you'd think that would lay off now!' We're reminded of another discomfiting fact: the dying can also be very funny. Bragg is metaphorically holding Potter's deformed hands through his life story like the best clinical historian, like a truly sympathetic psychiatrist more interested in the human reveal than the academic niceties of pathology. Potter's despair at the destruc-tion of the NHS is overt; his love and pride of the achievements of the Nye Bevan-era transparent. He has a near Old Testament vitriol at the abused concept of 'community care' that he sees as a free market 'solution' to psychiatric care by putting the mentally ill out on the street.

Potter is interesting too on vocation. He's proud to admit he has one; he's no longer ashamed. This too should chime with many care-workers. Why be embarrassed about it? Bragg gets him to talk about his father with great sympathy. This is what the dying want to do – talk about what they love, what they've loved. But there's also his wisdom that glorifies in smashing rose-tinted glasses when looking at the past. He argues that we should look on our earlier lives with 'tender contempt', recognize our mistakes but without being too hard on our younger selves: we have lived and that's what counts.

A fascinating insight into palliative care comes when Potter calls his tumour 'Murdoch' as in Rupert, the Machiavellian newspaper magnate. Potter's anger is focussed on what still matters to him – a pity at what he sees as the venal corruption of his country, its language, and the commodification of everything. Potter is still raging, Dylan Thomas-like, against the dying of the light. Many people we meet in the clinical arena of the dying are like him and we should watch this video and remember that.

Before talking about evil and the devil, Potter takes a moment out to seek pain relief. Bragg helps him unscrew the hipflask. He knocks a slug back in what might be the bravest thing you'll ever see on video. Doctors, nurses, carers, patients, can all benefit from its viewing. Potter is revealed as human, not a *thing*, something he wrote about again and again and wrote against – the reification, the commodification, of people. Humans turned into *things*.

The interview finishes with Potter celebrating his GP and he names him – Paul Downey – who 'gently led me to a balance of pain control and mental control where I can work'. He says he's serene and knows he's going to die. He's confident he can go out with a fitting memorial. The whole watch is devastatingly inspirational. Bragg raises a glass to him as the lights dim.

2

COMMUNICATION SKILLS

ANRI SALA

You're a junior physician on the night shift admitting patients, getting their histories, starting treatments, and now dawn has broken; you're tired, exhausted, but you still have to tell your bosses about the new cases. You crowd around a bed with the notes and then you read what you've written down: 'This man was complaining of chest pain saying it was going down his left arm and so I diagnosed new onset angina.' Your boss asks the patient to go through his story again, describe the pain he had. And then you're gob-smacked when the man says he hasn't got *any* chest pain. He now says he has a tummy ache. He should have been admitted under the surgeons. You've wasted everyone's time. Was it your fault taking a poor history? Or has the patient misled you unwittingly?

An everyday event for care workers: the mutability of truth. Anri Sala has much to teach students and carers, indeed patients themselves, about the tricky nature of reality: what we think has happened, what we think we have done or said. Sala is an artist from Albania, and his *Intervista (Finding the Words)* (1998) is a work that every healthcare student might benefit from seeing (Godfrey, Obrist, & Gillick, 2006). It lasts an excruciating 26 minutes.

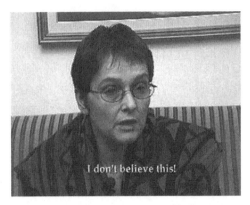

I don't believe this!

Anri Sala: *Intervista (Finding the Words)* (1998).

We see Anri with his mother, Valdet, a woman in her early fifties. He wants to show her some film footage he's obtained of her as a younger woman, some film taken about 20 years previously during the dictatorial Communist regime of Enver Hoxha. So we are watching a video of people watching a film. Unfortunately, there is no sound in the original footage. His mother laughs at her previous self, her dated fashions. This is a piece of pleasant nostalgia for her. She has no memory of the event.

Anri then goes to some length to rectify the silence of the film in order to restore meaning to the images. He visits a school for the deaf and gets one of the teachers, an expert in sign language, to read his mother's lips to see what she is saying in the old film. The images of his 50-year-old mother in the here and now are then intercut with shots from the classrooms where kids are using sign language with one another.

We return to the Sala living room where Anri asks his mum to look again at his newly *revised* version of the old black and white film, this time with subtitles. There are many ways to confront your mother and her 'truths' but this, we might argue, takes the proverbial biscuit. She then watches her younger self again (longer hair, no glasses) as she spouts ideological nonsense as detailed in the words now rolling below her image. Stuff about revisionism and Marxist-Leninism in support of the dictator, Hoxha. In the here and now of the post-Wall era, she's in complete shock faced with this truth. As with our patient and his disappearing chest pain, now located in the abdomen, she's changed her history. *I never said that*!

Unreliable historian. How many times have you heard that phrase on a ward round or read it in case notes? An old consultant boss of mine would always counter that the real unreliable historian was the person taking the history. Anri's mum disputes she said any of the statements she clearly made, as evidenced by the old videotape.

'I don't believe this!' She's absolutely adamant. She gets angry. What is even more interesting is that it's not the ideas per se that she objects to but the language she uses, the syntax. It isn't hers; it belongs to Hoxha's regime. Valdet is confronted with the awful truth in the here and now that she was being manipulated in the past: manipulated to distort language in the Orwellian style of 1984 and Newspeak. The film finishes by showing more recent footage from Albania taken at the time of a catastrophic collapse in the free market. Both far left and far right ideologies have been a disaster for the country. Valdet is left frightened about the future. We are all very aware of how the media can distort the truths of the present.

Valdet concludes the video by saying that she thinks her generation has passed on to Anri's the ability to doubt and that 'you should always question the truth'. This is the crux of the video, a credo you might argue for both artistic *and* medical practice. Today we are presented with scientific 'truths' at medical and nursing schools, told them on ward rounds and at the clinic, but we must – at all times – be prepared to challenge these if the evidence is weak. How strong is the evidence base? Informed scepticism is essential to the scientific method. We have seen all too many disasters (Thalidomide, the opioid misuse scandal) happen because healthcare workers have not asked enough questions.

Sala's video thus studies denial and belief, the fallibility of memory, and, I'd propose, could be a powerful tool in teaching carers, medical and nursing students, about the insidiousness and sheer power of denial. The video could also be recommended to those dealing with patients who have challenging beliefs, for example, those who reject advice informed by serious evidence-based medicine. This has become an increasing problem during the collective global experience of COVID-19 denial and those promoting anti-vaccination propaganda.

Anri Sala shows us that history with a capital H is akin to medical history taking and has absolute parallels too with medical historiography. The developments in medicine are an on-going dialectical process; as with all forms of science, we come up with hypotheses and test them to destruction. The examples of bad thinking in medicine are legion. Medicine, like history, is not finite. There's always more to learn. We used to think duodenal ulcers were due to stress and not *H. pylori.* We get things wrong and must always question and have doubts.

Then there's the question of personal trust. We must trust our carers. Anri's video asks even tougher questions on the nature of trust. Anri Sala was faced with a real problem – could he still trust his mum knowing that she was parroting the language of a totalitarian state when he was a kid? Can you trust a doctor or a nurse after they've got it wrong? How do you rebuild trust?

GILLIAN WEARING

Gillian Wearing is interested in trust and truth telling. One might imagine medical history taking as a secular form of confession. There are all sorts of reasons why someone may be reluctant to tell the whole truth when medical staff ask them about symptoms. For example, it is well known that carers working in the genito-urinary clinic have their tasks cut out for them when they do contact tracing. Gillian Wearing is interested in confessional truth telling. She knows much of our time is spent wearing masks; masks to conceal our inner truths – this is what her art is about.

Patients wear metaphorical masks: they might appear unconcerned, stoic, but underneath they are often in a state of what Nabokov (before his own bronchoscopy) called 'controlled panic'. Medical workers wear invisible masks too: we cannot express our true feelings of pity in many cases. We show 'controlled pity'. We stifle the urge to break into tears. No one wants, or expects, a doctor or a nurse to collapse in a heap bawling when they're meant to be looking after us.

Wearing's work gives us a 'judgement-free space', a term that might equally apply to medical practice. Our job is to cure people, help people, palliate people: it is not our role to judge. Wearing has a physician's distance from her subjects. She's a great listener: attribute Number One for the ideal medical practitioner.

Her *Confess All On Video. Don't Worry You Will Be In Disguise. Intrigued? Call Gillian Version II* (1994) is a work that says what it does on the tin. We see a variety of people individually, each wearing disguises – fake beards, wigs, faces distorted with Sellotape – as they relate a story that has been, up till then, private. We don't really know if they are telling the truth or embellishing their story, as with our collective experience in medical history taking. One of the major challenges in clinical practice is how to distinguish between *genuine* symptomatology and those individuals who have either invented or exaggerated complaints. Wearing's video highlights this dilemma. She's made other videos with a similar theme such as *Trauma* (2000) and *Secrets and Lies* (2000) where individuals, again disguised with masks, tell, as to a psychiatrist or a psychologist, what has harmed them. Not a stretch then to argue that watching these may be of real value in psychiatry training.

One of the most important communication skills is the ability to stay silent and let the patient do the talking. Wearing highlights just how difficult keeping quiet can be in her video *60 Minutes Silence* (1996). Here a large group of policemen and policewomen are seen in uniform. They are in three rows, the front are seated, the middle stand, the back group are on a platform. They stare at the camera and fidget, make the noises of movement. At the end of the film, one lets out a loud yell of relief. Why has Wearing used the police? We are reminded of their key statement: *You have a right to remain silent*. Patients do too. Like the medical profession, the police know that silence, when appropriate, can lead to proper detection, diagnosis, confession and ultimately, one hopes, a form of healing.

Patients (and medical staff!) can be dangerously self-absorbed. Wearing's *Dancing in Peckham* (1994) is an interesting example of such behaviour. We see her in a shopping mall listening to a personal stereo, indifferent to the passing crowds. She's jiving away; she's in an utterly different world from those around her. Wearing anticipates the many narcissistic self-portraits available minute to minute on social media platforms like TikTok and Instagram.

Wearing reminds us too of the importance of masks and the ubiquity of embarrassment, the reluctance to admit to habits that may be bad for one's own health. Her work could be used to teach health workers about ambiguity in patient histories and the pain of traumatic confession, for example, in genito-urinary medicine and HIV care. Then there are the ambiguities around compliance as in 'why I haven't been taking my tablets/my insulin', a regular issue for GP's, physicians and, in particular, diabetologists and endocrinologists.

Wearing is also interested in moments when the mask slips. We see this in the clinical situation, perhaps most often, when we have to deal with the inebriated, the intoxified. *Drunk* (1997–1999) is, predictably enough, a three-channel, 23-minute video of people who've drank too much alcohol. We watch them slur and stagger, watch them bob around, see them argue and spark out. Making an assessment that a patient may have drunk too much is not always easy and Wearing's video gives us a distanced view of how people look after overindulging. Wearing has also made works that interrogate identity issues relevant to healthcare that will be studied in Chapter 6.

CHRISTINE BORLAND

Communication skills are now actively taught at medical schools. Christine Borland has made and curated works that specifically address the challenges students face when talking to patients. Her exhibition *Communication Suite* (2008) was designed for the Medical School at Glasgow University. This was held in a part of the school where ten pairs of rooms are used to train students. Each pair consists of a dummy consulting room and a seminar room linked with closed-circuit surveillance cameras of the sort pioneered in art by Bruce Nauman – an American artist to be discussed in Chapter 4. Actors play simulated patients and the medical students are faced with scenarios they are likely to encounter on qualification and practice. The scenarios often feature exercises in breaking bad news – 'tell this patient they have cancer' – and so on. Exams for higher post-graduate training (e.g. the Royal College of Physicians PACES) often feature such 'stations' for assessment in communication skills.

The actors, tutors and peers observing the student, provide feedback on the 'performance' as to how they have 'performed'. Particular attention is given to body language, eye contact and obvious examples of empathy. Borland is particularly interested in the performative aspects of these interactions – care workers are usually naturally empathic but on occasions this needs to be 'acted'.

Her series *Simbodies* & *Nobodies* (2009) featured six digital videos of simulated bodies being made, the likes of Resusci Anne. Borland documenting the process and so we see the hot fake heads of Airway Larry and Choking Charlie cooling and condensing under glass domes after they've been pulled from their plaster and silicone moulds. Borland has also made a trilogy of videos – *SimMan* (2007), *SimBaby* (2008) and *SimWoman* (2010) – that film each 'doll' in an eerie light that heightens their spooky verisimilitude to real humans. It's the breathing movements of the chest that get to you ....

Borland is also fascinated by the possibilities for miscommunication and how this might be avoided. She organized specific workshops for medical students *and* students from Glasgow School of Art to explore issues of communication and miscommunication; this was interdisciplinary practice in action. This too can be seen as an early example of how video art can inform medical practice.

Communication Suite also involved works by other artists such as *Îles Flottantes* (2008) by Douglas Gordon (2006), another Scots artist discussed later. We see a garden pond scene worthy of Monet disturbed by several skulls bobbing on the surface of the still waters: a reminder of the great *vanitas* art projects, that in the midst of the beauty of life we are in death. The video *AAA-AAA* (1978) by Abramović/Ulay was also shown where both performers face one another and say 'ah' as with lung auscultation. Here the *aah* sounds become longer and louder as if in a face-off, a fight. Their mouths get wider. Their pitches rise in caterwauls of noise and they get hoarse. They could be in pain. The performances are anguished but fake – a reminder that everyone can act.

TIKTOK 1

But acting can only get us so far as regards education. One of the strengths of new social media platforms that use video clips is that they can highlight the real, the unmediated (Comp, Dyer, & Gottlieb, 2020). Here's a TikTok video entitled *You Have Cancer* in eight parts where @careersdoctoruk, an oncologist, takes us through the process of breaking bad news. He outlines ethical issues, how to listen and be empathic. He says: 'Don't say things like *I know what you're going through* – because you don't.' What he says is thoughtful and entirely appropriate to the situation. There's little doubt that he is an empathic doctor himself, but his series raises an important question: can empathy be taught? Or is it an innate quality in an individual? Can video artworks develop empathy in carers towards those who suffer from stigma?

3

STIGMA, TRAUMA, AND THE BODY'S VULNERABILITY

This chapter examines how artists have studied our inherent physical frailty, as well as violence and heightened emotional states such as despair and sadness. We will also look at issues such as self-harm, and other physical and psychic challenges that are daily events for healthcare workers. We will review how video addresses stigma and how it might help those who suffer from stigmatization.

Sitting in the waiting room of an accident and emergency department, sitting in an orthopaedic outpatient clinic looking at the fractured, you might ask yourself: *do we ever learn?* Instagram and TikTok feeds are a feast of idiocy – as with endless numbers of skateboarding stunts that end in disaster, the parkour pranks gone wrong. How many traumatic events do we have to go through before learning basic lessons about gravity, about the danger from knives and guns? Can artists help us to understand our tropism towards risk and self-harm? And can they do this with humour?

RODNEY GRAHAM

Vancouver-based Rodney Graham was one of the funniest artists who used video until his untimely death in 2022. His *Vexation Island* (1997) is a colourful nine-minute production. In one sense, we might see it as a parody of glossy advertising or mainstream cinema.

Set on what appears to be a paradisiacal Caribbean island, we first observe the iridescent cobalt waters of the sea lapping on the deserted white sands. We cut to a palm tree stirring gently in the breeze and then recognize a shipwrecked sailor (Rodney himself) sleeping under the said tree. He's dressed in eighteenth century garb wearing a jabot and a red waistcoat. A stunning yellow and blue macaw parrot waves its wings as it perches on a barrel near Rodney's feet. You're thinking of Robert Louis Stevenson, treasure, *yo-ho-ho and a bottle of rum*.

The camera then pans up to the undersurface of the palms, and we see a coconut dangling from one set of fronds. Cut to Rodney again. He could be a pirate; he bears a strong resemblance to Johnny Depp with his moustache and locks. Is that a bruise on his forehead? The waves lap in gently, the sun shines down from a bright blue sky; nothing threatens, this is the holiday dream beloved of a million travel agents. But then – uh oh – there's another close-up of Rodney's brow. That's more than a bruise – it's an old clot. He's been hit! Has another pirate assaulted him? Has he been robbed of his booty? Or is there a Man Friday out there defending his property? Is Pirate Rodney a drunk who's overdone it on the rum? Is he ... (gulp) ... dead?

We now note that Rodney's head rests on a chest. His eyelids twitch and he wakes. He squints into the sun then gets distracted by the parrot waving one wing in the direction of the sea. He sits up as if to quiz the bird, then the camera gazes up again at the palm fronds. The parrot persists in making the pointing gestures with one wing. Rodney stands up and we see him from behind; we note – tick – his piratical pigtail. He scans the horizon, looks around through 360 degrees and settles his gaze on the palm. He looks up and shakes the tree; he's hungry and thirsty; he's seen the coconuts. His shakes intensify and a cusk falls down in slow motion towards the camera lens; it hits Rodney right on the bonce. The parrot glances over knowingly. Rodney the pirate now falls, again in slow motion, a Keaton-esque pratfall in all its amusing pathos. He's spark out and we are back to where we started.

You get knocked down and you get up again. We're in Nietzsche's world of everlasting recurrence; time in a loop. We're in the A/E department. Graham's work is thus an amusing one-liner about consciousness and unconsciousness but also a parable about accidents and how they will always happen. We never seem to learn, or find it very difficult to learn. I can imagine *Vexation Island* going down well if it was shown on flat screen TVs in minor injury A+E waiting rooms: it could function both as a tool to cheer up the mildly traumatized and as educational parable.

Graham's other works often deal with identity, and he has a Sherlock Holmes-like interest in the signifiers of clothing and habits such as smoking and drinking. He's a diagnostician of sorts and his observational skills are, like Holmes', worthy of study. Close looking is another lesson from art applicable to clinical practice. Clues to pathology are literally staring us in the face – the tattoos that might hint at underlying Hepatitis B, the nicotine stains on fingers pointing to an underlying bronchial malignancy, and so on.

Graham's practice reminds me of one of my first clinical lessons from a boss prone to hoary old tricks. He was teaching us about glycosuria and how the ancients could diagnose diabetes by tasting urine. He held a sample in a plastic urine container, unscrewed the lid and dipped a finger into the yellow fluid. He then popped it into his mouth and said 'Sweet!' We looked on in horror as he handed the plastic bottle to one of our group and commanded: 'Go on, try it!' As soon as my fellow student made to taste the urine the boss stopped him, raised a hand and said:

> *Now, listen up and remember this. Clinical observation is the key to medicine. If you were looking carefully you would have seen that I dipped this finger* (here he waved a cheeky middle digit) *into the urine but tasted* this *one.*

The licked index finger was now pointing upwards in our faces. Giving us the finger in a Rodney Graham kind of way.

BAS JAN ADER

Not every story has a happy ending. Bas Jan Ader's father was a Dutch resistance hero who saved Jewish lives and was executed – shot – by the Nazis. How do you live up to that as a son? Impossible perhaps but it might inspire you to make an impossible kind of art. Your subject will be 'the impossible', and, like Chris Burden who we will discuss later, you can show how fate is set against us. You can show *how* we are vulnerable. We are programmed to get ill, we are programmed to die. You can show how we fall.

Ader's video works are not a million miles away from the endless sequence of risky clips mentioned earlier that we see on Instagram and TikTok, where young people make skateboard leaps, BMX bike jumps and parkour acrobatics. Indeed another Dutch artist – Ger Van Elk – had himself filmed doing other idiotic albeit gentler challenges as with *The Flattening of the Brooke's Surface* (1972) where he uses a paddle to smooth out the ripples on a stream. We might read this work as a parable about never-ending clinical tasks such as checking INRs at the warfarin clinic or dampening fluctuations in blood glucose levels in diabetes. Ader's stunts are also funny but performed without irony – he really is testing gravity, testing fate.

We love to test out our bodies, as A/E and orthopaedic surgeons will testify after one of their rescue missions in theatre. Here's Bas Jan carrying a chair and climbing onto the top of the roof of his house in Los Angeles – what's he up to? This is *Fall 1* (1970): we see him balance on the eaves like Steve McQueen's tightrope walker and then position the chair. He sits on it then tilts forward only to fall to the ground. He looks unhurt but chastened. He's the real Man Who Fell to Earth. Gravity will get us all. At some point we all fail, we all fall.

Broken Fall (organic) (1971) sees Bas Jan hanging by his arms from a tree swinging above a burn. His hands clutch at a thin branch. You know either he or it are going to give way but you're not sure which or when. Tension builds and then his arms let go, he can't take any more, he's dropping, there's a splash and then he's under the water. His actions again recall Buster Keaton: his fall is both comic and tragic at the same time; it's our lot in life, whether we're the patient or the carer, to be left hanging until the eventual drop.

And here he is yet again with *Fall 2* (1970) where he's cycling along a canal path in what looks like Amsterdam. He passes a humped-back bridge and then careens off the road only to end up in the water. He's telling us that slapstick is real; we all end up in the soup, down the drain.

How might one react to this depressing realization? Tears? *I'm Too Sad to Tell You* (1970–1971) is a powerful silent film of Bas Jan crying for some unknown reason. He brushes his hair away from his face with one hand, clutches at his brow and wipes his eyes. He does not meet our gaze. At one point, he seems on the cusp of bawling. You're reminded of Carl Theodor Dreyer's great silent movie *The Passion of Joan of Arc* (1928) where the actress Renée Jeanne Falconetti weeps copiously. We are beyond verbal language here. Ader can't tell you what's upsetting him in words. Here is loneliness caught in a short video. Is he crying for his parents? His lost father or the lost Jews? Maybe he's weeping for us all? Perhaps he's crying just for himself. He knows he will fall and fail again and again. This work could have an obvious role in teaching us about the grieving process or even potentially of use to grieving people themselves in a sharing capacity that says 'you are not alone'.

Bas Jan's final work is *In Search of the Miraculous* where he set off in a small boat to sail the Atlantic. He tells his wife he might be back in three years. But he disappears and the myth begins. His boat was found wrecked off the Irish coast. Bas Jan was never found; he's gone to the great unknown. The myth survives. Was it all a stunt? Is his death a fake? Has Bas Jan really gone?

Another way of considering Ader's doomed quest is to compare it to that of the medical scientist: he, and they, are trying to find what cannot, as yet, be found. As his brother says Bas Jan was 'trying to see over the horizon'. His works are metaphors for exploration, the Romantic strive for more knowledge, enlightenment. And all the while facing the ever-present risk of failure.

Mistakes. All medics, all carers, all patients, make mistakes. We need to think on our mistakes, analyse them, talk about them and prevent them from happening again. Ader's work on mistakes, on gravity and falls, has proven an inspiration to many other artists. Pipilotti Rist, mentioned elsewhere on works that deal with woman's issues, is seen falling and near drowning in *(Absolutions) Pipilotti's Mistakes* (1988). Geriatricians tasked with the prevention of falls may be interested in other Ader works clipped in Gavin Maitland's documentary on the artist: *In Search of the Miraculous* (2007). We see Bas Jan make yet another fall, this time from another chair; he's trying to balance on two of its legs. There's always a tipping point: there's always a split second where the trick might come off.

Maitland's documentary also shows other artists making videos of 'deliberate' accidents. In *Neon* (2003), Monsieur Moo shows a seated figure wearing a hood sat outside while objects crash down on their head. And we see Tsui Kuang-Yu being hit on the back of his skull by a large object in *Eighteen Copper Guardians* (2001). Friedrich Kunath shows himself doing fake falls in various public street scenes in *After a While You Know the Style* (2000). And Guido Van der Werve goes the whole hog and takes artistic self-harm to the limits by having himself run over by a car in *Nummer twee* (2005). But what might be the ultimate risk to the self? What about getting shot at?

CHRIS BURDEN

Grainy footage for sure but what we see in *Shoot* (1971) still shocks. Chris Burden's video is an eight-second clip of the artist being shot by a friend with a 0.22 calibre rifle. Burden is on the left of the screen wearing a white T-shirt, his arms bare. To his right, a friend (Bruce Dunlap, a Vietnam draftee) aims a rifle at him from 15 feet away – as if he were in a firing squad – and shoots. Burden is clipped in the arm and staggers forward, clutching his wound: end of artwork. How can this be art? And if it is what can it tell us as carers?

In another video, this time a documentary made decades later, we hear the older Burden, by this time an established and much respected artist, explaining something of his intentions. The Vietnam War was at its height when *Shoot* was made. As Burden says – 'you saw a lot of people being shot on TV every night'. And so the work is not only about violence and damage to the body per se but also about violence on the TV – the nullifying, distancing effect TV has. Burden was making a critical video *about* video, about TV. We recall Marshall McLuhan's role as Cassandra, how the medium of TV can be the message, the war-like message being: *Shoot people!* Burden, we might argue, is making the cartoon nature of TV violence real again. Burden makes a martyr's gesture in order to make a political point, a psychological point about desensitization, something that may happen to all of us through watching too much TV, too much video....

Shoot clearly highlights issues about violence, the bystander effect, the reality of guns and what harm they can do. Accident and emergency physicians, public health officials, can relate to the lessons of this video that basically says: 'Don't muck about with weapons. Don't do it kids. They hurt people. They kill people'.

Generation Z is well aware of this issue. For them, 'the prevention of violence is ... a high priority' with gun control being a key issue (Katz, Ogilvie, Shaw, & Woodhead, 2021).

Burden has also talked about his attempts to control fate, or rather as he says 'the illusion that you can control fate'. Again a day-to-day lesson in A/E departments, in medicine in general: *you can't control fate*. Burden made other works that undermine TV, that critique this form of video. He bought advertising time and placed bogus adverts. Some of these were humorous as he put himself in the line of artistic greats from the past. Another shocker aligned to *Shoot* was *TV AD* (1973) where he is seen crawling over glass for a couple of seconds. There's much debate about Burden's work as regards self-harm and whether or not these videos should have been banned. Can such works encourage others to repeat crazy stunts?

TIKTOK 2

This in turn raises contemporary concerns about social media platforms such as TikTok that are predominantly used by the young (Alaniz, 2022). A recent (and greatly publicized) case in the UK highlighted the dangers of vulnerable youth watching self-harming videos. *The Independent* newspaper reported a possible 20 deaths of children in an 18-month period linked to a 'blackout' challenge (Sarkar, 2022). As with similar stories following the arrival of radio, movies and TV in the past there is a seriously negative side to progress.

TV MEDICAL DRAMAS

Burden's insistence on the real has implications for those watching medical dramas on TV. These are extremely popular and often quite convincing but do not capture the lived reality of Burden's actions. TV medical dramas major in voyeuristic incident and quick resolutions. They may encourage an interest in working for patients (a good thing) but all too often the actual demands of the job far outstrip the excitements seen on the TV. TV dramas avoid the tedium of holding a retractor, skirt the demands of exasperated individuals tired of waiting. There's the real risk that the glamourization of the medical profession on TV sets up unrealistic expectations in both patients and future carers. And unrealistic expectations can lead to a breakdown in trust....

VITO ACCONCI

Speaking of trust Vito Acconci's *Security Zone* (1971) is the perfect metaphor for the carer/patient relationship as regards its being the near ultimate in placing confidence in someone, someone you don't know. This is a work on vulnerability at its most maximal. One person is chosen to act (dually) as a guard and/or a potential opposition party – we remember that carers and patients are in a kind of opposition given that one is well, the other unwell. Acconci is the Other: the person who has to place trust. Acconci, like a patient, has ambiguous feelings about this 'guard', this putative doctor or nurse. As he says in explanation – 'the guard is a person who's moves I don't fully trust'. Even the most trustful of patients will have moments of hesitation, moments of questioning.

Acconci, to an extent like a patient, is blinded: he's made to wear a blindfold. His ears are plugged, and his hands are tied. Again, like a patient, he may not be able to hear what's being said, he may misunderstand explanations from the carer. He or she feels bound, helpless. Acconci is spun around by the guard and made to walk around an abandoned pier surrounded by water. He's under the control of the other person, the guard, in the same way that patients often feel when undergoing complex treatments.

Many patients will recognize Acconci's vertiginous sense of confusion when we are made to listen to medical language. The carer, in Acconci's instructions for the work, 'determines how to use the trust I am forced to have in him/her'.

There is the possibility that the relationship will improve but there's always the threat it could go wrong; Vito – like Bas Jan Ader – might end up in deep water. The clinical encounter is always a source of danger; it can degenerate into confusion, conflict. Acconci's video reminds us that there's always work to be done to gain trust because of our ongoing vulnerabilities.

REBECCA HORN

Ongoing trust becomes even more of an issue in chronic illness. The vulnerability of the body to long-term sickness is highlighted by Rebecca Horn's video *Scratching Both Walls at Once* (1974–1975). We see the artist in a room with bare white walls. What's she going to do? She walks away from the camera and holds her arms out, and we immediately see that she has long talon-like extensions tipped with pencils attached to her arms. She walks towards the windows while dragging the long pencils against the walls making her mark. She's saying 'I count, I will make my mark' despite her disability.

Horn had known significant periods of being bed bound that led to a year's stay in a sanitorium. The work is therefore a metaphor about the unwieldy nature of disability, the limitations of bodily constraint and how we might fight this. What can we learn from this work? It's lessons are similar to those that feature in many of Oliver Sacks' stories on neurological disability: we need to imagine what it is like to be immobile if we are caring for the bed bound, we need to speculate how we might manoeuvre ourselves if we have a fractured leg, or a severe multi-joint arthropathy.

JENNI-JUULIA WALLINHEIMO-HEIMONEN

This Finnish artist has osteogenesis imperfecta and her short video parable *Battle of Scarcity of Resources* (2017) features a cute red squirrel behaving selfishly toward a tiny model of a figure in a wheelchair and is a witty and pithy reminder of the discrimination and violence against people with disabilities. We need to think of the prejudices such sufferers face from the uncaring well. We need to think about stigma.

STIGMA AND VIDEO

Stigma might be defined after Erving Goffman's key book on the subject as 'the situation of the individual who is disqualified from full social acceptance'. Goffman, in his preface, highlights clinical studies on facial deformities. He talks of three grossly different types of stigma:

1. Physical deformities.

2. Societal perceptions around 'blemishes of individual character' inferred from a history of 'mental disorder, imprisonment, addiction, alcoholism, homosexuality, unemployment, suicidal attempts, and radical political behaviour'.

3. Tribal stigma of race, nation and religion.

One might add a fourth – the 'invisible' – that it to say those who suffer stigma from a majority yet to significantly admit to the existence of such prejudice.

Those who do not depart negatively from what Goffman calls 'the particular expectations at issue' he calls 'the normals'. Video art has much to teach 'the normals' in the caring professions about those branded with stigma, those who suffer from exclusion. Essentially what video artists do here is render us *considerate* in an inconsiderate world; they help us imagine what it is like to be 'othered'. Video artists put us in the shoes of the afflicted.

'To see oursels as ithers see us': as Robert Burns wrote in 'To a Louse'. This is what art, and in particular video art, can do. This is what carers must do. We must be benevolent to the stigmatized. This is the job of the doctor and the nurse: to 'soften and ameliorate' the pain of the sufferer. It is a short step to view those with a stigma as, in Goffman's words, 'not quite human'. From there discrimination begins, we reduce life chances, and the road leads on, inexorably, to atrocities. And words, everyday language, can speed this process: words like *spastic, cripple, moron, cretin*. Words that can be abused, words often used to promote stigmatization.

Stigma towards people with mental illness is a particularly persistent problem (Angermeyer, Matschinger, & Schomerus, 2013) and public attitudes are often inaccurate (Pescosolido et al., 2010). Up to 54 per cent of respondents on one study thought people with schizophrenia are violent or dangerous (Stip, Caron, & Lane, 2001). Similar views may even be held by healthcare providers themselves (Knaak, Mantler, & Szeto, 2017), as such stigma often leads to discrimination and exclusion. How might we try and improve this situation? Video has been argued as one way to reduce stigma (Mitchell, de Lange, & Molestsane, 2017).

One recent innovative study has looked at the use of participatory video (PV) to reduce stigma (Whitley, Sitter, Adamson, & Carmichael, 2020). They looked at three workgroups of people with mental illness all of whom made videos and then had these disseminated locally to target groups. The study thus examined the feasibility of using PV in people with severe mental illness *and* made an assessment of viewer impressions and their subsequent subjective impact.

According to the authors, a PV project can be defined as a group of marginalized people coming together to script, film and produce bottom-up educational videos about shared issues that affect them. The group has complete editorial control over the content and themes. Videos can be made in a documentary style or feature the experience of a single person; this latter is known as Digital Storytelling. Key to the process of PV is the subsequent showing of the videos to a community setting in order to educate and, hopefully, enable change. The videos are thereafter shared on social media platforms and can be accessed at www.radarmentalhealth.com, www.youtube.com/user/recoverymentalhealth

Locality is important because there is the suggestion that this increases, in the study's words, 'watchability, affinity and resonance'. There is evidence that this may be more effective than the use of celebrities or actors (Stuart et al., 2014). We will come back to this idea when we look at the work of the artist Candice Breitz.

The authors go on to stress that PV has the potential to 'confront stereotypes and illuminate day-to-day "behind the scenes" realities of recovery' – as opposed to the negative impact of TV news reporting on mental ill health that tends to stress stories around crime and violence. There are some excellent Twitter accounts that highlight recovery and the ongoing challenge of mental ill health such as @charliersmith1.

Given that our current digital lives mean large numbers of people now obtain information from social networking platforms and streamed videos there is a strong argument, say Whitley et al., that mental health advocates should 'harness these innovative visual methods to reduce stigma'. They stress new efforts 'must be based on solid research and scientific evidence'.

Three workgroups in three different Canadian cities were recruited for the study. Professional videographer-facilitators were hired with teaching experience to help with scripting, filming and editing. Each group made a video and then screenings were organized to three target demographics: students and young adults, health and social service providers and the general public. Overall 1,542 viewers were reached. A questionnaire was used to assess impact of the videos.

The questionnaire was brief and could be adapted for similar future studies looking at physical ill health and even, as we will discuss later, exposure to art videos dealing with health issues. Simple questionnaires maximize response rates and allow ease of interpretation. The research team in Whitley et al.'s study had two items reverse coded to reduce bias. The questions were:

1. The video changed my attitudes towards people with severe mental illness for the better.

2. My understanding of stigma has not increased after watching this video.

3. The video led me to better understand recovery from mental illness.

4. The video had little impact on my outlook towards people with severe mental illness.

5. My behaviour to people with severe mental illness will change for the better in light of this video.

Viewers would then rate the amount they agreed with each statement using a 5-item Likert scale ranging from 'strongly agree' to 'strongly disagree'.

A total of 1,104 completed the feedback questionnaire and aggregated responses showed a moderately positive impact on viewer attitudes to mental illness. There was a consistently stated view that the videos were educational and informative. In particular there was the impression that the videos made 'an ideal introduction to the issues and challenges associated with living with a mental illness'. The words 'relatable' and 'real' cropped up frequently when describing the videos. Generation Z are known to place great emphasis on the 'relatable'. Some viewers also described how the experience helped them 'reframe their perspectives' as regards mental ill health, with some adding that it changed their 'behaviours towards people with mental illness for the better'.

The study concludes by saying there are two key findings:

1. That PV is a feasible 'anti-stigma intervention'.

2. That the data suggest that the videos positively affect viewers and can be an effective means of stigma reduction.

The authors argue that these results have policy implications given that 'stigma reduction is a key target for mental health policy in various jurisdictions globally'. The authors also suggest further routes for research as with formally measuring the impact of the videos 'longitudinally through repeated measures with validated instruments'. To their knowledge, this study is 'the first large-scale multi-site project examining the feasibility and impact of PV for people with mental illness. Can we use the lessons of this chapter to study the impact of video art?

CANDICE BREITZ

Using a variant on the questionnaire above, I would propose a similar study following a viewing of Candice Breitz's video *Love Story* (2016). The purpose would be to see if exposure to this work has an impact on healthcare students' attitudes to the six individuals in the film, all of who have suffered trauma or stigma of one sort or another.

The work is in two parts – in one hall we see six screens (each with headphones attached) where we can sit and listen to the person talking to us, telling their story. The individuals are all refugees and so we hear Sarah Ezzat Mardini escaping from the destruction of Syria; Jose Maria Joao, a former child soldier denied education in Angola; Mamy Maloba Langa, a victim of sexual violence from the Democratic Republic of Congo; Shabeena Francis Saveri, a trans rights activist from India; Luis Ernesto Nava Molero, a highly educated Venezuelan political dissident; and Farah Abdi Mohammed, an atheist from Somalia. Each of these individuals is confessing to us, the listeners, as with telling a medical history at a clinic. We're reminded of Gillian Wearing's earlier works. As with clinical encounters at outpatients these people are placing trust in Candice Breitz and we, the audience.

In a neighbouring hall is part two of the work, or part one should you choose to watch this initially. The artist does not dictate which part to attend first – it's your choice. On a single screen we see, alternately, two famous faces: the Hollywood actors Alec Baldwin and Julianne Moore. Both talk to us and, if we've paid attention to the words spoken by the refugees in the neighbouring room, we immediately recognize that it's *their* narrative, not the actors.

'It was a small inflatable for nine or eight people ...' the words of the young Syrian refugee in halting but excellent English are smoothed out by the warm Californian tones of Moore. Baldwin's husky voice, his hand gestures, recall those of an action hero – the words though belong to Jose the child soldier. The Hollywood actors act out the words they've learned and we see them make many different facial gestures as they repeat the traumas of the six people in the other room. They wince and glare, stare at us intently at times, come near to tears. We hear how they stress certain sentences, how they can shift vocal tone for dramatic effect.

'Some of the most pressing issues of our time came into the limelight only after Hollywood actors and actresses performed certain roles.' So says Moore, quoting one of the refugees, but confusingly, confoundingly, sounds like she's talking about herself. Baldwin goes on to say 'I'm sure there are millions and millions of actors who really sympathize with refugees. We're human beings just like you'.

What is Breitz trying to reveal here? First and foremost: how actors and actresses dramatize, how we believe in them, how we are convinced. And that this belief may be in stark contrast to what may be our first reactions to the refugees themselves. What might these be? Unacknowledged bias towards those with the stigma of exile: accents that we may strain to understand, appearances that are out with our own Goffmanesque 'normative' experiences. This is what Brietz confronts us with – in some ways, we might argue what we're experiencing here is just another day at the clinic listening to new people telling us their story. Do we have empathy with them? Do we believe them? Do we trust them? Do they trust us?

Breitz's work shows us that the manner in which a story is told has a huge influence on our ability to empathize with a sufferer. We may be more moved emotionally by the professional actor than the *real* person. We live in a society that arguably values mediated experience – cinema, the simulacra – over the real thing, the real truths, that are all too often too difficult to deal with. We crave entertainment, as with French writer and philosopher Guy Debord's talk of 'the society of spectacle', the world of mass media manipulation. Our need for entertainment may be to the detriment of dealing sympathetically with the *actual* sufferer.

My contention is Breitz's artwork may have a directly positive impact on the attitudes of carers in training. This is a video that forces us to listen and pay attention to the real rather than the performative and to try and acknowledge the difference. The artist made the work after witnessing the mass movement of migrants to Berlin in the mid-2010s. She's interested in what is called 'the attention economy'. In the West, some people get the attention (currently the Ukrainians under attack from Russia) and some do not – as with, say, Yemeni children being bombed by Saudi Arabia.

A similar attitude prevails in medicine: certain conditions, certain specialties (cardiology, say) grab much of the medical 'attention economy' to the detriment of the non-glamorous but essential services like rehabilitation medicine and elderly care.

The mixture of people in Breitz's work tells us that anyone can be a refugee and by extension anyone can fall ill, can become stigmatized. Breitz's choice of individual, the six people she chose, deliberately subverts notions of the stereotypical exile.

TIKTOK 3

There is any number of short video works on TikTok, Instagram and other social media platforms that highlight stigma, disability, suffering and resilience. These, we must assume, empower the sufferer. Take this everyday example from TikTok @shaniesfight where we see a young 23-year old in a hospital ward wearing oxygen prongs. She's got a funky topknot and quickly tells us she's awaiting a double lung transplant, maybe for long-term cystic fibrosis. She points to her ECMO lines and then asks us to enjoy her presentation about the technique. An upbeat rap soundtrack announces 'I'm about to show you what I'm made of'. We see images of her with her boyfriend, shots of her posing like a model outside with her machine. There are backdrops of palm trees and Californian-style architecture. 'I'm way too strong. I'm an icon' sings the rapper. The sheer forcefulness of the young woman's bravery strikes the viewer. Thousands have seen her videos.

You can only be humbled seeing these. This is anecdotal evidence of their effectiveness and both carers and patients could benefit from watching such short productions. The distanced nature of the videos encourages us to witness such trauma. But then there's Polish trauma … and Jewish trauma.

KATARZYNA KOZYRA

Many contemporary Polish artists make work about trauma (not a surprise given the tragic history of their country) and the vulnerability of the body. Katarzyna Kozyra filmed herself during sessions of chemotherapy for Hodgkin's disease and posed *a la* Édouard Manet's *Olympia* (1863) for a series of photographs. She's personally aware of the indignities of illness, the trauma of anti-cancer medication and its horrendous side effects. We see her post-chemo with her hair loss and her black choker and bright flowers as with Manet's original. Just as Manet confronts the male viewer, the male gaze, Kozyra does this too but she *also* gazes back at us, the healthy, the well – Goffman's 'normals' – challenging what we might call 'the well gaze'. Her work forces us to look at an ill person, consider what the illness and treatment have done to their body, and think about being unwell, helping us to understand the implications for the sufferer.

Kozyra has also filmed the poignant effects of ageing with a video called *Women Bathhouse* (1997) taken in the Gellert baths, Budapest. This was shot with a hidden camera and we see women on six channels washing themselves. We might argue these are some of those 'invisibly' stigmatized as proposed earlier: the inevitable 'invisibility' that comes with ageing. There is no disguising the effects of age in the bathhouse; this is not the body beautiful as depicted by Ingres or Manet, or that shown regularly in contemporary woman's magazines obsessed with perfection. Many of the women in the baths are elderly and overweight or cachetic. Knees are knobbly; arthritic gaits predominate. Kozyra has said she wanted to 'show women as they really are, not touched up, not fake'. The scene is in no way eroticized; this is the body as failing entity, a sad thing; again the fate that awaits us all. Images from the Holocaust are obviously conjured but the showers here jet water not Zyklon B.

A follow up work – *Men's Bathhouse* (1999) – saw Kozyra infiltrate the men-only space using make-up and a prosthetic penis. She found that men are

> *more relaxed ... women try to show themselves in a better light ... they're more graceful on the whole. Men couldn't care less. They scratch their ass and their balls in public too ....*

There's always room for Rabelaisien humour as we stare at our lot. Given the current debate around access to toilets and gender it's interesting/humorous/alarming to hear that Kozyra felt 'terrified' when she did this, worried sick that her prosthesis would fall off.

Watching both videos offers an important lesson to care workers. There is intense pressure to mix patients on wards due to bed shortages as a consequence of government cutbacks. The dignity of many patients is thus bypassed and poorly considered. As a result, many of the people we are trying to care for endure yet another level of discomfort and indignity. As Kozyra's work illustrates men often behave in an uncouth and undignified manner, sometimes unintentionally, sometimes hilariously. But many women really don't want to see this and deeply resent the idea of mixed-wards. Are such managerial decisions, imposed by politicians, steps in a dehumanization process? Is this part of a political drive that ultimately leads to further savings, further indignities? We recall the slow degradation of human rights under the Nazis after they came to power in 1933. Which brings us to ...

MIROSŁAV BAŁKA

The ultimate example of the body's vulnerability – and humanity's greatest trauma – is the Holocaust. Do doctors and care workers need to know the workings of the Holocaust? Absolutely: Robert Jay Lifton's (1986) book *The Nazi Doctors* tells us in chilling detail how the medical profession was deeply complicit in killing the mentally handicapped and mentally ill long before the establishment of the death camps in Poland. Doctors and nurses were subsequently a key element in the organization that exterminated millions of Jews, thousands of gypsies, gay people, religious and political dissidents. Without knowledge of how the Holocaust was perpetrated the medical profession is doomed to repeat the enabling of similar atrocities. The video artist whose work centres on issues about the notorious crimes committed on Polish soil is Mirosłav Bałka.

Carousel (2004) is a video taken at the site of the death camp at Majdanek. The work is projected onto each of the four walls of the gallery space. What we see is vertiginous, an experience not dissimilar to those suffering from acute labyrinthitis: a fast-circling shot that destabilizes us, that deliberately sets out to disorientate us and give us the merest glimpse into the horrendous world that the camp prisoners endured before being murdered.

Another video – *Bambi (Winterreise)* (2003) – shows a snowy winter scene that could otherwise look like a cutesy example of Christmas kitsch. But again, there's dirt behind this daydream. Deer playfully frolic around a field, an image of the life force going on despite the history of the site. This is Auschwitz, and we now see the horizontal lines of barbed wire. The deer forage for food and we are forced to remember the ill-clad inmates, freezing in the cold. We can imagine them seeing the freedom of the deer, their ability to gallop away, to escape.

Bałka's *BlueGasEyes* (2004) is unusual in that the two video screens are placed horizontally onto the floor. We see two flames from a standard gas cooker – two blue circles accompanied by the hiss of gas. An ordinary enough image, even beautiful and hypnotic to contemplate, but Bałka is making us remember how this simple technology was used to kill huge numbers of people.

Was resistance even possible? Despite ludicrous odds against them a handful of Jews did escape. Bałka's work *B* (2007) teaches us that resistance, even in tiny gestures, may be worthwhile, may make – like Rebecca Horn's work – a mark. We see a TV screen with what appears to be an inverted letter B. It's snowing outside. The 'B' is part of the word 'Arbeit', part of the sign over the gate at Auschwitz – part of the cynical message 'Arbeit Macht Frei': work sets one free. Look again at that 'B': it's upside down. The prisoners charged with making the sign slipped in a subversive message. Do not believe that this place is a resettlement camp. Do not believe everything is in order. Here disorder rules; here truth – like this B – is inverted.

The lesson here via video art for the medical profession is that we must speak out when faced with more contemporary acts of evil, whether we're confronted by venal pharmaceutical companies as outlined in Patrick Radden Keefe's (2021) book *Empire of Pain*, or faced with anti-science nonsense such as those who decry vaccination policies. The indifference of the medical profession kills. And, sadly, there is always the potential for doctors and nurses to become active killers themselves. The profession did not teach this crucial lesson at medical schools in the late twentieth century. It must now. I argue here that video art is one way to do this.

4

NEUROLOGY AND PSYCHIATRY

Look carefully at many admission notes, and you'll no doubt read the phrase 'grossly intact' or some such under central nervous system (CNS) examination. In real life, this means the doctor has seen that the patient's arms and legs appear to work normally on a cursory viewing, and that the patient's vision and hearing seem normal. It can't really be called an examination as such but time constraints – *there's ten patients waiting to be seen in the corridor, doctor* – mean that this may have to do when dealing with a teenager suffering from, say, severe acute asthma. We can make a reasonable assumption that their neurology is, for the immediate present, okay. But what do we mean by 'grossly intact', by 'normal'? We begin this chapter by studying a video artist whose work in part exemplifies the examination of 'normal' neurological function.

BRUCE NAUMAN

'Examine this man's gait': a standard instruction in practical exams for doctors in training. You're asked to watch someone with Parkinson's disease shuffle along – in medical jargon, he's festinating – chasing after his centre of balance. Or else we might observe someone else with the wide circumducting swing of the leg seen in a patient who has had a previous stroke. One of my own personal ways of teaching medical students on neurology was to ask them to *mimic* certain neurological gaits. They would watch me impersonate – and then copy – the idea being that not only would it help them recognize certain neurological conditions as a spot diagnosis but also give them some, even minor, insight into the reality of having to live with such a disability. Students thus get an idea of the incapacity, the sheer difficulty, of living with, say, the stamping gait of someone with peripheral neuropathy, or the radical imbalance that results from cerebellar lesions with their wide swerves and lurchings. Which brings us to Bruce Nauman.

Nauman is one of the most-renowned American artists of his generation. There's a consensus opinion that he's the Samuel Beckett of contemporary art; his works often appear deceptively simple but require detailed unpacking. Many of his works are video productions and not a few feature gaits and the strangeness of being an upright organism that walks. Physicians ask patients on a daily basis: *let me see you walking*. They would do well to study such Nauman works as *Walking in an Exaggerated Manner around the Perimeter of a Square* (1967–1968) and *Walk with Contrapposto* (1968). What are we seeing here? In the former Nauman is seen barefoot slowly pacing a chalk line on his studio floor. It's an endurance test of sorts; he's testing his balance. You're reminded of childhood games of tic-tak-toe. His neurology appears 'grossly intact'. The younger Nauman does *not* have the neurological disabilities we might be used to seeing from neurology training videos. And that's the point: we are watching normal neurological function under duress, something we take for granted and rarely study – a normal man walking. Nauman is training us in observation.

He updates the latter work for the new century as *Contrapposto Studies* (2015–2016). Here he's striking the classic Renaissance pose seen when we shift our balance mid-walk, our weight transferring from one foot to another. Decades have passed since his initial version; this is a different, older, Nauman dealing with a new and more challenged sense of cerebellar control. He's in his seventies now and has had a colostomy; we can see the bulge of his stoma bag through his T-shirt. We're now being asked to look again at ageing and the body's frailty.

Frailty and its assessment are major concerns for care workers. Geriatricians and occupational therapists in particular would benefit from seeing Nauman's work. As said earlier: *let me see you walking*. We ask the elderly to get up and walk as part of our assessment for discharge. We watch the frail and judge them as fit or unfit for home, in the exact same manner as we watch the older Nauman.

CHRISTINE BORLAND

There are gaits and there are gaits – some are distressingly pathological. Duchenne muscular dystrophy is a rare severe X-linked recessively inherited condition that causes serious gait issues. Boys are thus predominantly affected and lose muscle bulk in the thighs and pelvis that in time means they cannot stand straight. By age 12, most cannot walk properly. There is no cure although gene therapy holds out some hope for the future. Life expectancy is currently around 26 years. Neurologists and geneticists can tell you the facts but how might an artist give us an insight into the everyday reality of this condition?

Christine Borland has made a video – *Endless Walk* (1999) – that features an animation projected onto two corners of a room. Most of the time you enter the space there's nothing going on – just a bare white minimalist area, what critic and doctor Brian O'Doherty labelled the classic white cube. But then something happens in one of those corners. We see a cartoon video, a line drawing features a child crawling, a child with Duchenne muscular dystrophy. The crawl is not normal. Firstly, you realize the child is not a toddler, they're much older. Secondly, they have what neurologists call 'Gower's sign' – they have trouble getting up from a lying or sitting position and thus 'walk' with their hands clutching their feet. The animated figure moves across the screen then disappears from view. A few minutes later it reappears on the other corner only to disappear again, then reappear in the first corner after another void of time.

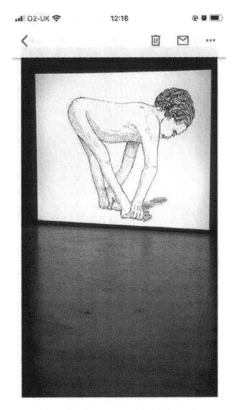

Christine Borland: *Endless Walk* (1999).

The duration of the walk, the crawl, is thus accentuated, stressed for our observation. What we're being asked to do by the artist, forced to do even, is to contemplate the time it takes for someone with Duchenne's to 'walk' from here to there in the room. It's a work that asks for deep empathy with the sufferer. The video thus has a strong emotional and educational impact, illustrating as it does the severity of the condition. *Endless Walk* could be used in paediatric and neurological teaching to underline the impact of the disability for carers.

JACQUELINE DONACHIE

Moving on to another genetically inherited neurological condition, we now encounter Jacqueline Donachie's work. Donachie is another Scottish artist trained at Glasgow School of Art; she's interested in myotonic dystrophy. This condition was diagnosed in her family in 1999. Her sister and brother have it, she herself does not. Donachie says that the trauma of the familial diagnosis made her want to address this via her art. She collaborated with the geneticist Darren Monckton to do a project called *Tomorrow Belongs to Me* (2001–2006) that features video work. This contains interviews with clinicians, scientists and patients, and hones in on 'anticipation' a genetic concept that explains why the condition gets worse as the generations grow. Donachie's own niece and nephew exhibit this progression.

Donachie is particularly interested in the fact that the families themselves had long known about this phenomenon but many scientists were reluctant to accept this given the controversies around eugenics and the aforementioned crimes of the Nazis, their policies of euthanasia for those with inherited conditions. It goes without saying that Donachie's work is illuminating to carers involved with genetic abnormalities.

Another of Donachie's videos is *Hazel* (2015). This features a split screen with two sisters (five sets of siblings in all) and is informed by ethical issues and ethics training. One sister has the condition, has the gene: the other does not. In one case, there are three sisters. The work stresses the diversity, not only of the condition but also of the identity issues regarding facial appearance and we hear: 'These are things we tend not to ask about in the clinic…'.

The actual geneticists caring for the patients have noted this interesting aspect of the work and thus we have a definitive case, definitive evidence, of an artwork that has influenced the *carers* themselves. Dr Mark Hamilton of the West of Scotland Clinical Genetics service is quoted as saying:

The effect of the silent sister – a range of different women from the general population – reminds us that the affected sisters are equally diverse, and encourages us to look beyond the superficial similarities of the disease and to see the individual.

And again:

> *Certainly I think this has made me much more mindful of*
> *identity issues in my approach to patients with Myotonia*
> *Dystrophica.*

There's a powerful poignancy to watching *Hazel*. One sister describes the effect the condition has had on her face – the obvious ageing, the ptosis (drooping eyelids) – while on the other screen her unaffected sibling looks at the camera in pitiful silence, we can't *not* compare the two people, can't *not* imagine the dynamic between the two, the sheer unfairness of life's genetic lottery. Inside they are thinking – why has this happened to me and not her? Why has this happened to my sister but not me? The clinician's eye, the viewer's eye, goes back and forth between the two faces in comparison. We think too of society's demands on women and the ubiquity of media insistence that women be perfect in appearance, be beautiful. What if you've no say in this? What if your agency, in this regard, is stolen by a neurological condition?

A more recent video, *Pose Work for Sisters* (2016), features Donachie herself and her own sister, balancing on white plinths. This is partly a tribute to another Scottish artist, Bruce McLean, who performed an earlier work parodying classical sculptural poses. The discrepancy in the sisters' ability to adopt positions,

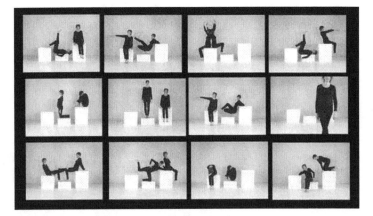

Jacqueline Donachie: *Pose Work for Sisters* (2016).

their flexibility, could be seen as biology's cruel differencing, but we can also argue that it is a profoundly empathic work, showing as it does the impact of the condition. There are, as Donachie says, deep similarities as well as marked differences in families as a result of myotonic dystrophy.

Donachie makes art that is directly involved in scientific research. Hers is an art that can be directly used in patient and carer education. Her work in depth, complete with patient and carer interviews, can be consulted via her PhD and the publication 'Tomorrow Belongs to Me'.

DOUGLAS GORDON

Winner of Britain's Turner Prize in 1996 Glaswegian artist Douglas Gordon makes video art inspired by cinema and film. Some of his earliest works, such as $10ms^{-1}$ (1994), featured appropriated footage from old medical libraries. As with Christine Borland, Gordon is interested in the ethical issues raised by such artefacts. Watching $10ms^{-1}$ is, initially, a confusing experience, even for someone medically trained. To those without a medical education, it must seem baffling. What we see is slowed down black and white film projected onto a wide screen. From the grainy quality of the print we can tell the images are from the distant past, the beginnings of cinema. We see a man, naked apart from shorts, on a floor. He's trying to get up but his legs don't seem to work. He's using his arms to raise himself. Has he Duchenne's muscular dystrophy?

On first view, some would be forgiven for thinking this is some kind of modern choreography, perhaps a dance piece by the likes of Merce Cunningham. A closer examination shows that those legs we may have been thought paralysed (is he a paraplegic?) can actually move, can obviously abduct and adduct. And this isn't Gower's sign, this isn't muscular dystrophy, because in other shots his legs seem to work normally. He has muscle bulk but cannot get up. He's fighting against gravity – as in the title – 10 metres per second per second. What's the diagnosis?

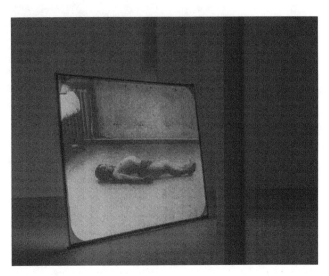

Douglas Gordon: *10ms⁻¹* (1994).

The man is a war veteran, and the film was made some time after his demobilization. He's back from the trenches of the First World War. He has some kind of shell shock, what physicians call a 'non-organic' or 'functional neurological deficit', what used to be called 'hysteria'. Neurologists have long had to distinguish between organic neurological deficit due to disease, an often incurable or actual anatomical disruption and non-organic dysfunction, symptoms that are fundamentally psychological and potentially treatable/self-resolving.

Physicians can watch *10ms⁻¹* today as something of a learning aid in distinguishing between organic and non-organic pathology, an issue that remains live in neurology and as relevant today as in the time of Charcot. We might cite here a paper on Oliver Sacks' (1984) experiences outlined in his book *A Leg to Stand On* (Stone, Perthen, & Carson, 2012). The authors reappraise Sacks' story and conclude that he was suffering from a functional paralysis. And we are reminded too that Charcot's use of the tendon hammer to elicit or not elicit reflexes was used to challenge French soldiers thought be 'malingering' in an effort to avoid call-up against the Prussians.

Watching the patient struggle to rise can be seen as tragi-comic – his movements are vaguely ridiculous, near slapstick in their incoordination, their denial of the reality of normal neurological limb function. This could be a Buster Keaton clip but it's not laugh out loud funny: it's profoundly sad and profoundly private. The man's psychic trauma from the war has led him to deny the power of his own legs: he doesn't want to go back to being mortared.

Even more explicitly troubling for today's carers of the neurologically or mentally ill is *Hysterical* (1994). This is an older newsreel footage, where we see (one assumes) a group of be-suited, mustachioed Edwardian era doctors handling a woman with an undiagnosed functional disorder (Debbaut, Gordon, & McKee, 1998). She throws herself around: some will find this, as we say today, 'hysterically funny' and yet the footage has a powerfully charged sense of sadness – the pity evoked by unenlightened times now, thankfully, long gone. But 'hysterical' conversion syndromes are still very much with us, as contemporary neurologists attest (Stone, Hewett, & Sharpe, 2008).

Gordon's interest in conversion syndromes may be seen as partly literary/historical, partly clinical, but perhaps more importantly the work asks us a deep ethical question: Who shot this original footage and why? Was it purely for educational purposes or was there an element of ghoulish entertainment at work? This is a question that could be asked of Gordon's own motives: his work majors on doubling and the doppelgänger; his is a particular Scottish interest in opposites, a worldview often referred to as 'Caledonian anti-syzygy'. We recall that in the past patients with mental illness have been viewed by the public as a spectacle in places like Bedlam. Did the patients in *Hysterical* and $10ms^{-1}$ give truly informed consent to this invasion of privacy? Did they know the film would be stored? How would these patients feel if they knew this footage would be used in the late twentieth century as 'art'?

Gordon has also spoken about homeopathy and how his family were interested in the concept and, as with digoxin, 'a tiny amount of herbal influence could cure, or kill, the body'. There's an argument that as an artist he functions, in some of his videos, as a kind of doctor pointing at an underlying diagnosis he can't yet name. He's clearly interested in perception and memory in other works and in particular 'where perceptions break down'.

Another of his 'hysterical' works is *Trigger Finger* (1994) featuring more non-organic pathology. Is there an artist alive who is more interested in hands and what they can do? You don't need to be a hand surgeon to find his hand works fascinating. Gordon cuts off his circulation at the wrist with cords; imitates finger gangrene with tattoos; makes obscene gesturings; appropriates R. L. Stevenson's famed palmar black spot. He's made a series of works that feature fingers, hands and hand gestures such as *A Divided Self* (1996) and *The Left Hand Doesn't Care What the Right Hand is Doing* and *The Right Hand Doesn't Care What the Left Hand is Doing* (both 2004) that deal with duality in the individual – that anti-syzygy again. He also refers to R. D. Laing's (1960) book on schizophrenia, *The Divided Self*, a topic we will return to in the work of Luke Fowler.

Perhaps Gordon's most famous work is *24 Hour Psycho*, a drastically slowed down version of Alfred Hitchcock's most famous movie, a work that, in its insistent use of *delay* gives carers and future patients a real understanding of fear: fear being perhaps *the* most important impact on the individual of illness; its amelioration and dissipation being the crucial role of the carer.

ERIK VAN LIESHOUT

More everyday neurological events are the subject of Erik Van Lieshout's video *René Daniëls* (2021). Lieshout's work features a fellow Dutch artist who suffered a devastating brain haemorrhage back in 1987. René has been left with a severe expressive dysphasia but he still paints. What we see are two artists in a most unusual form of communication that effectively revolves around the words 'yes' and 'no'. Van Lieshout remains patient and relaxed throughout his interactions with Daniëls. They sit at a table outside with paper and crayons. Daniëls cradles his affected arm. They walk around town and chat with some schoolkids who seem both amazed and confused when Van Lieshout tells them that Daniëls is actually quite famous.

There are scenes with Marleen Gijsen, Daniëls' carer, who doesn't fuss over him but helps when he needs assistance. There's a refreshing everydayness around their interactions; the video is devoid of sentimentality or easy grabs at pity. Daniëls and Gijsen have to get on with their lives. Van Lieshout is determined to show that despite Daniëls' disability he can and does function as a working artist. His receptive capabilities appear to be not significantly impaired and neither is his artistic expressiveness as regards his drawings. Only his verbal language skills, his actual ability to get words out, is devastated.

Daniëls uses other means to communicate: he smiles a lot and he frowns a lot. There are his ubiquitous hand gestures – waves and thumbs up and so on. We think of Douglas Gordon's fascination with hands gesturing, waving, conducting. But there are limits to the interaction between the artists; ultimately Daniëls' world remains something of a mystery to Lieshout. What Daniëls can say he predominantly, pre-eminently, says via his painting and drawing.

In my view this is another work that should be required viewing for all healthcare workers in stroke medicine, which means all physicians and GPs. Those trained in occupational medicine will see how Daniëls' artistic activities give him a grip on life. Watching the interaction between Daniëls and Van Lieshout is informative because we see care delivered in an impassionate manner; he and Gijsen give Daniëls proper loving care. Care that needs time and substantial amounts of patience, both sadly in significant short supply in the hard-pressed health delivery systems of today.

PIERRE HUYGHE

Cutting-edge technology can inform artworks about neurological function. Pierre Huyghe is a French artist. His *UUmwelt* (2018) uses MRI scanners and computer networks; it's a piece he's made in collaboration with neuroscientists. Several LCD screens show videos of what appear to be an ever-changing and constantly fast-flickering sequence of images that never become entirely resolved. Some look like they might be insects, some are ill-defined animals – *was that a dog?* – and some might even be faces. Before you can be sure of what you're seeing the image has mutated into something else.

We're told what we're seeing represents an interpretation of human brain activity through data captured by an fMRI scanner following an individual's exposure to visual material and verbal descriptions. These images on the screen have been produced via 'a deep neural network' system developed by the Kamitani Laboratory in Kyoto, Japan. They can apparently turn these data into a collage, a reconstruction of what the mind 'sees' (Shen, Horikawa, Majima, & Kamitani, 2019). The work thus aims to capture what the brain is 'seeing' when asked to think about a specific object. In turn, we are thus looking at images from someone else's brain in constant flux with our *own* brains trying to decide – is that a chicken or an insect? In the immediate instant after we question what it is in front of us it has gone. So we are thinking, and trying to interpret, an image said to be that of what someone else has been thinking about, has been trying to 'picture'.

Perception in all its complexity is what we are being asked to consider: what is abstract and what is real. We look at abstractions – that pattern in a marble table that looks like a face, those cloud shapes in the sky – and try and make sense of these, we work through what we may or may not recognize. The tease in Huyghe's work is that we are asked to look at someone *else's* mind running through its image bank in search of recognition – just as we are doing the same thing with their 'pictures' in front of *our* eyes. We are all trying to make sense in our different ways of what is in front of us. The work then is a metaphor for our individual condition as regards receptivity and its unlimited variability. And this metaphor applies to both our appreciation of art *and* scientific observation. In this sense the work illustrates and even mimics the task of a radiologist: pattern recognition and close looking. And of course radiologists don't always agree with one another ....

The title of the work – *UUmwelt* – refers to a term used by the German biologist Jakob von Uexküll. He talked of the *umwelt* – our environment or 'surrounding world' – that describes the experience of being *in* the world as *specific* to each biological entity. That added 'u' in Huyghe's neologism of a title might be understood as a *un-umwelt*, that is to say a means of bypassing of our own individual responsiveness and thus have an open-ness to other ways of seeing the world: how a fly or a dog might view their surrounding worlds. Huyghe's work can thus also be seen as another metaphor for the use, even the meaning, of art. Again: *to see oursels as ithers see us!*

Huyghe's work is of clear interest to those training or delivering neurological and radiological care. I saw the work with a neurologist friend and we talked for hours after about its evolving meanings, its implications for the self.

LUKE FOWLER

And speaking of the self, Luke Fowler's *All Divided Selves* (2011) is a 93-minute video about the life and work of psychiatrist R.D. Laing. Laing's *The Divided Self*, published in 1960, questioned previous attitudes to schizophrenia. Laing was no fan of ECT, lobotomies and the like. Contemporary psychiatrists have subsequently discredited many of Laing's ideas but his work illustrates the ongoing dialectic in the medical world about schizophrenia and its aetiology. Fowler is interested in the unresolved, the ongoing questioning of Laing's knotty legacy. The Scots psychiatrist was something of a Jekyll and Hyde figure, charismatic but said to be prone to violent outbursts: more of that Caledonian anti-syzygy.

Fowler's video is a collage that vacillates between the critical responses to Laing's radical 'anti-psychiatry views' and his later international media success. Laing became a household name and embraced a fame that brought its own problems – a particularly pertinent issue today for many young doctors who embrace celebrity TV appearances or YouTube/Instagram/TikTok slots as 'experts'. There is a flip side to what might be considered as advertising – a practice regarded, indeed taught, as unethical in my medical school days. For those who embrace self-advertising in medicine the accountability bar is raised significantly and reputational damage can occur if misleading claims are made via public forums. Many professional organizations – the Royal College of Physicians (2021) for one – have codes of conduct that outline the risks of social and video media platforms. Fowler's work could thus be used in teaching psychiatrists and other medical staff as to the perils of media exposure and fame. The work can be hired out via Lux online.

TIKTOK 4

Type 'Multiple Sclerosis' into the TikTok search engine and within seconds you can listen in to individuals like @annaleahart who quickly go through their own presenting complaints. She had symptoms that initially didn't make sense, that weren't listened to by her carers. Her advice is sound: 'keep talking'. She tells us about her numbness and tingling in one limb, then how this switched sides to the other leg. Then she talks about falling over 'like I was inebriated'. All classic features of MS.

Back to the search engine and look for 'temporal lobe seizure'. Under you can hear Addi, a young person talking about their seizures:

At the beginning the seizures present as really really extreme déjà vu, like almost a doom déjà vu feeling. I avoid certain movies and songs – they might not trigger a seizure but they make me feel like I'm going to have one at a particular moment.

As with Anna Lea's MS video there is a striking immediacy to such evidence. We are witnessing Addi talking about movies that set of a temporal lobe seizure – a discussion we might wait months or years to encounter via traditional medical teaching.

As said this is a random selection from TikTok. The sheer volume of clinical material out there on the platform is astonishing. As with Jacqueline Donachie's (2016) work on Myotonic Dystrophy there are several patients on TikTok with MD demonstrating, for example, how difficult it is to open and jar and so on. We assume each person posting has given their consent to appearing in a public forum given that they themselves have done the filming, pressed *send* to the world. Of course a proportion of these *may* be fakes. But many look very real and are shot *live* with little or no rehearsal. Such videos must be considered clinically useful given they appear as immediate and impactful as someone describing their previous experiences of ill health in a lecture hall.

Consent and insight as regards social media platforming becomes even more problematic when we type/search for mental health conditions. Does this individual know the full implications of what they are doing if they post details of their own issues with, say, schizophrenia? We're reminded of the earlier work on PV – participatory video. Support groups for such people suggest PV may well be useful and further research on the value of video here seems essential.

5

ABJECTION/GASTROENTEROLOGY

Degradation and disgust; piss and shit and blood. That's the bottom line in healthcare (pardon the awful pun). Being a patient, nursing and caring for a patient, means getting messy. Cleaning up: it's a dirty job but someone's got to do it. Effluvia: the humiliation of being reduced to an abject vomiting wreck, a diarrhoeal disaster, is a common lot of the ill. We've all been there but how can video help us understand abjection? Julia Kristeva (1982) has written on the horror of abjection, how it undermines identity and being; how it screws up the programme, the routine. The abject, for Kristeva, is

> *a frontier, a repulsive gift that the Other, having become alter ego, drops so that the 'I' does not disappear in it but finds, in that sublime alienation, a forfeited existence.*

A forfeited existence – that's having a bout of D and V all right. Her writing has been a powerful influence on a generation of video artists.

This chapter will study artists fascinated by the gut. By extension it's also a review of work about effluvia – and how, laid low with GI upset – we become abject. The hope is that having seen these works gastroenterologists and those caring on gastro wards may develop a better insight into the problems of patients with these issues. Abjection is surely a strong feature of admission to a gastro ward. Not for nothing has the gastro unit in our local hospital been nicknamed 'Beirut', a place where disasters happen.

Let's cross Kristeva's frontier where 'the clean and the proper ...
becomes filthy'.

PAUL MCCARTHY

Paul McCarthy's videos feature ketchup, HP sauce and mayon-
naise firing out of squeezy plastic bottles; for these read blood, shit
and semen. Read spurting, ejaculating: fluids leaking and flowing
out of control. His work is astonishingly transgressive and has the
visceral impact of being soaked from head to toe by a geyser of
variceal blood. Or the stench after walking onto a ward where
some poor patient has just unleashed a torrent of melena stool.
Why is McCarthy doing this to us? One explanation he gives for
his wild works is that they are 'some kind of symbolic expression
of my own fears'. Professor Kristine Stiles thinks one of the princi-
pal metaphors in McCarthy's work is: 'the body as threatened and
denigrated, unable to find its way into the knowledge of its condition' (Rugoff, Stiles, & Gioni, 2016). Think of the last time you
were unwell with gastroenteritis following food poisoning – you
know you're not well but you can't do much about it, you're helpless, you have no clue what organism, what toxin, is attacking you.

  'I think my work deals with trauma, my experience of trauma,
physical/mental trauma/abuse.' So McCarthy continues in an interview with Stiles. 'My actions are visceral; I want it to be visceral.'
He's mirroring our own personal experiences of trauma in order
that we, his audience, gain some insight, any insight, into our true
condition, the often sad and tragic condition of being human.
McCarthy wonders if his art can function as some kind of a vent:
'I was thinking about venting trauma, and that art could act as a
vent'. He's punning here:

> *Vent: noun 1. An opening that allows air, gas, or liquid to
> pass out of or into a confined space. 2. Release or expression
> of a strong emotion. 3. The anus of a lower animal. OED.*

Do his videos work as a vent? Everyone will have their own take
on his actions; many will find his videos horrible and, not unrea-
sonably, feel disgusted and walk away. Others will stay rooted,

appalled that McCarthy is telling us visually, as Beckett does in his writings, that this is our lot as humans: *get used to it.* What appears on screen – as with the ketchup smearings and outpourings in *Pinocchio Pipenose Householddilemma* (1994) and *Bossy Burger* (1991) – will remind some of the aforementioned variceal bleeds, the true horror as gouts of blood erupt, a fountaining out the mouth of a cirrhotic patient. Can you prepare yourself – as a doctor working on a gastro ward – for such a calamity? Maybe not, but McCarthy's visuals give you some idea of what's in store for you when some unfortunate cirrhotic's varices blow.

The curator Ralph Rugoff calls McCarthy 'the master of the taboo-smash'. He goes on to say that we are witnessing the defilement of the body, albeit in a theatrical performance, one that mirrors the catastrophes of real life, a life that can be seen as 'hellishly dark and terribly funny'. There's something to *laugh* at here? Rugoff is right – medics and healthcare workers use gallows humour all the time – Rabelaisian japery as coping mechanism. We know, as Rugoff goes on, that McCarthy's 'ketchup is blood, but at the same time we always know that it is ketchup' – reminding us of the horror movies discussed in Steven Schlozman's (2021) book in this series, *Film.*

Rugoff continues: 'At times, (McCarthy's) regressed behaviour evinces an excruciating autistic poignancy'. What Rugoff calls 'our unease with spontaneous emissions' occurs because they remind us of our mortality – we are, to quote another Scottish pop singer – Davy Henderson – just beef and electricity. Eventually our plug gets pulled.

What appears in McCarthy's work to be faecal incontinence is only liquid chocolate and his use of ketchup as simulacra asks how *real* can simulation be? When healthcare students see mock-ups – as per Christine Borland's *Communication Suite* – can they take them seriously? Isn't there (always?) a wide gap between the real and the acted-out? Isn't it the case that actual live apprenticeships with real people, real bodies, will always out trump fake re-enactments no matter how much sauce and make-up you use?

This in turn leads to another thought – the *distancing* effect of video. Video as teaching material appeals to only two of the senses – seeing and hearing. We cannot touch, we cannot smell, we cannot (thank God!) taste. Video, like all art forms that deal with medicine, can only get so close to the real, the actual.

McCarthy goes for the gut: as Dean of Yale's School of Art and critic Robert Storr points out he's in the tradition of the nineteenth century cartoon satirist James Gillray. McCarthy is a pessimist telling us we're in the swamp. His cloacal obsessions in turn force his critics to chomp on gastroenterological metaphors, an appropriation of medical language. Hence we read the artistic director Massimiliano Gioni saying some of McCarthy's work appears 'gluttonous, bulimic and insatiable'.

Have you ever had an enema as prep for a sigmoidoscopy? No? Then as a patient pay attention to McCarthy work: he's giving you the heads up that it's not going to be nice. And if you're a carer this is what you'll be dealing with when faced with the bedbound, the incontinent. Fluids, lots of them: scary, smelly, sticky fluids. Storr admits that McCarthy's work has had a profound impact on his own self and assumes that

> my preparedness for that effect identifies common ground
> at some existential level or in some of the inner chambers
> of the psyche where life's hard knocks are absorbed and
> processed.

You might have a similar experience after seeing a McCarthy video.

WIM DELVOYE

Here's a video on Vernissage TV, a channel that documents art openings; it features one of Wim Delvoye's *Cloaca* works. The clue is in the title. We see a queue of people in front of an enormous metallic tube that is the size of a large truck. It might be a reactor of some sort with its pressure gauges, its metallic sheen. Is it a distillery perhaps? Are the people here for a free drink? Some men in red T-shirts and blue overalls seem to be the technicians – they look like Super Mario. We learn that this version of Delvoye's series is called *Super Cloaca*. They chop up piles of vegetables and fruits on a table. The crowd mills around inquisitively. We get a glimpse of the back of the machine and see plastic bottles, connecting tubes.

Is it an engine of sorts? Some kids help the artist (himself dressed in that ludicrous Super Mario outfit) as he loads a small ramp with chunks of food, bits of banana, slices of carrot. These move upwards like a mini-escalator into the maw of the machine. From some angles, it looks like a giant cannon, a weapon. What will it unleash?

Shit. The machine makes faeces. *Super Cloaca* is a gut. Delvoye has collaborated with scientists to create an enormous artificial gut. This is only the most recent iteration of his idea. His first digestive machine was more open in structure and looked like a series of chemical experiments: six large bell jars sat on metallic tables connected by transparent plastic tubing. There's a set of ladders at one end where the mouth is. This is niche bioengineering. Delvoye says his work reminds you that you are an animal and in one sense his machines address our embarrassment over bowel function. He's asking us to marvel at what the gut does. To *not* be disgusted by it.

Trainees in gastroenterology, nurses on gastro wards and patients with significant gut dysfunction might learn a lot from seeing these works. The *Cloaca* project provides us with a fantastic and unique insight into the very complexities of gut function. For a group of scientists and an artist to create a simulated gut requires serious ingenuity. Delvoye talks of the pepsin and bile salts that are added to the mix as it churns along the chain of artificial stomachs, artificial intestines. It's not hard to be impressed at what this chain of chemical reactions represents, what the real gut does. Somehow evolution has provided us with this entire apparatus, concertina-d, compressed, inside our belly.

Delvoye also talks of his debt to Piero Manzoni, another Rabelaisian artist, a conceptualist who canned his own excrement, a gag on the capitalist commodification of everything. Artists have always been interested in everything human, even that which shames us, even that we can't see ....

MONA HATOUM

And what of our own invisible human guts, our own intestines? Mona Hatoum's *Corps Étranger* (1994) is a two minutes footage of the artist having an endoscopy, all sound-tracked by her own heartbeat as heard from Doppler echocardiography. Clearly, this is yet another image of vulnerability. We see the mucosal surface of her oesophagus, the lining of her stomach, the coarse folds of rugae. You might think of food: this is where it goes. You might even think of tripe – some of us eat stomach, cow stomach, with that carpet-like texture it has. Here is a glimpse of the hidden interior, Hatoum's insides that connect with the outside. The inside that is also the outside; there's a hole that runs right through us. The gut surface, like the skin, is our front-line, the border between us and the world.

There were interesting ethical issues in the making of this work. Did Hatoum actually *need* an endoscopy? Did she pay for one without any clinical indication? Did the gastroenterologist or nurse specialist who performed the procedure do it for free? If it was all done for art what would have happened if it had gone wrong, if she had suffered a perforation? Does this make the work a brave or foolhardy act? Didn't medics themselves once experiment on their own bodies? If they can do it, why can't an artist? Can we see the work as being of use to patients about to undergo the procedure? Perhaps. *Corps Étranger* says: 'Look at this – this is what your doctor will be seeing, this is what you look like, inside'.

Another great benefit of video – as form – is that we can make videos of our *own* reaction to video; we can film ourselves giving our own opinion on works of art. This is true of Hatoum's work on YouTube. A student called Meyke Werdmolder has filmed herself talking about *Corps Étranger* and she provides a neat, quick insight into the work. Her own explication could be used as an example of 'how to approach art about medicine' when teaching healthcare students. She points out that you have to enter a small cylindrical room to see the work, a kind of gut in itself if you like. We learn the footage of the endoscopy is actually projected onto the ground.

Meyke admits to feeling 'uneasy' when she first saw the work, a not unsurprising take from a non-medical individual. Medical workers need to be careful about recommending footage of procedures to patients – not all have hardened stomachs. Meyke understands Hatoum wanted to make a work about the invasion of the body, a violation in some respects of the body. She also explains that the title of the work is multi-referential. The inside of the body is foreign to us and the endoscope *itself* is a foreign body. And we are, in a real way, foreigners to our own bodies. Meyke also reminds us that Hatoum herself is viewed (by reactionaries) as a 'foreign body' given her status as a Palestinian Lebanese exile in the UK.

In her conclusion, Meyke says something of great value to patients and carers alike. To quote her:

> *The artwork gave me a different perspective on my own body, the self (that is myself). I now realize that the gap between what I know about the outside and the inside of my body is enormous and it forced me to look at my body in an unusual way, and that my ultimate private space is foreign to me.*

Meyke's short video essay is also a great example of how we might teach students to interpret video works for themselves. Her thoughts work in two ways as regards using video in medical education: firstly, we can say – look here, watch this viewer's explanation *after* you've looked at the video of the art work, *after* you've made up your own mind about the work and ask yourself if you agree with this other student's interpretation or not. This could be used as a preliminary to group discussion. Secondly, making a video of your own thoughts on a medically related artwork, or after dealing with a case, helps you to focus and tighten your conclusions, particularly before doing a live talk. We can create video self-portraits if you like: truly reflective learning. These have long been the practice of many patients on TikTok and we'll examine some more of these clips shortly.

MARTIN CREED

Martin Creed makes things without titles. His works are simple and are what they are – a crumpled ball of paper, a piece of blu-tac, a room where the lights go on and off; unsurprisingly there are those who wonder if he's being serious. Is this pile of chairs really an artwork? Are we being played? There's humour in his deadpan approach that skirts with the suspicion that he could be a charlatan. Creed is well aware of this risk in his strategy but his manner is charming and when he talks about his works he neatly combines the innocence of American singer Jonathan Richman (Creed plays in a band) with the ludic knowingness of Marcel Duchamp. Creed digs bold colours. He's into stripes. He works in sequences. He likes order. So why has he made a video, *Untitled Work No. 503*, where somebody vomits?

The background space to the work is completely bare in what might be a parody of Brian O'Doherty's (1976) standard gallery fixture, the white cube. We could also see this environment as a clinical area, a sterile ward perhaps. A young woman appears from the left. She's breathing deeply. Suddenly she puts a hand in her mouth and projects a stomach full of vomitus onto the bare floor. We hear her retch; we hear the shocking splash of the fluid. This is exactly what seeing someone being sick looks like and it always surprises, always worries. Aside from cases of obvious gastroenteritis (and bulimia/anorexia) vomiting is, for clinicians, a *bad* sign, a worrying sign. The doctor thinks – uh oh – does this person need admission? You're unwell if you're vomiting. I do not recall discharging *anyone* who was actively vomiting. So one of the benefits in seeing Creed's video is the *distanced* experience of observing someone who may be very ill. We note the dry spitting, the gasps for air.

Creed has made another version of the work (*Work No. 610 Sick Film*, 2006) where we hear the clack of high heels and see another young woman dry heave. She laughs at odd moments and says 'Oh, God'. Again you ask yourself – what am I looking at here? This girl seems to take some strange pleasure from the activity. Is she bulimic? Is she an actress? Does she have morning sickness related to pregnancy? This is yet another video that poses difficult questions of agency and consent.

For those with tougher defences Creed has even filmed people defaecating (*Work No. 660 Shit Film,* 2006). The transparency of these works is startling; these are not made for entertainment. Nor do they have the deliberately transgressive intent associated with the Viennese Actionists (more of whom shortly): there is no political motive at work here – these actions are for real. Creed's intentions remain poker faced. Again this work says to care workers: 'this is what this looks like, this is the real world – get used to it, you'll be dealing with it *a lot*'. If you do a cursory search on YouTube about 'different types of poo' you'll find any number of educational clips on 'what it says about your health'. We could even argue that these videos have replaced the old photographic images in standard surgical textbooks of steatorrhea stools, melena or the silver stool associated with carcinoma of the ampulla of Vater.

THE VIENNESE ACTIONISTS

Medicine has its fair share of shocking moments – that empyema which knocked you off your feet because of the vile smell of its pus or the carnage of major burns, the horror of traumatic amputation. It's doubtful we can *truly* prepare ourselves for the terrors to come but exposure to the work of the Viennese Actionists is one way of experiencing extremely distressing events via the distanced medium of the screen. As Schlozman has argued in *Film* there is a case for using horror movies as a means of 'creating empathy for conditions that seem extremely difficult to otherwise understand'. The videos of the Actionists are certainly horrific but an all-together different kettle of fish from, say, Hitchcock's *Psycho*. While I would doubt they are of any serious clinical use, I draw attention to them because they clearly influenced the other artists mentioned in this chapter addressing transgression.

The Actionists were Günter Brus, Otto Mühl, Hermann Nitsch and Rudolf Schwarzkogler. Their art is messy and, like that of McCarthy, involves fluids only this time they use *real* excretions. Their intentions were generally political – they wanted to shock the complacencies of an Austria still in denial at its contribution to the Holocaust. Carers and medical practitioners will recognize the carnage in their works, the uncontrolled nature of bodily (dys) function.

Filming your own abjection. The Actionists were ahead in this respect. Today this is not at all uncommon phenomenon on social media platforms. Filming your own trauma, your own stigma, in order to educate others about your pain.

TIKTOK 5

There are innumerable self-posted videos on TikTok featuring people with gastroenterological conditions – many of these talk of tips to heal ulcerative colitis and so on. Some of these are clearly unscientific and would be quite unhelpful. An argument can be made for the Royal Colleges (as upholders of standards) to ask some Fellows to view and grade some of these in terms of usefulness for patients. Give them a Kitemark if you like. Stoma care, for example, is brilliantly illustrated by @hiddenstitchesuk. She has over 3,000 followers and her swift, efficient, demonstration of how she quick changes her bag is educational, reassuring and quite inspiring.

6

IDENTITY

Considering a patient's identity is a key element of medical care. Get that wrong and you're in big trouble; the regulatory bodies deal regularly with such mistakes. This chapter examines how artists have approached this tricky area and contemplates the potential use of video works to expand the ability of carers to better understand/empathize with patients and their identities. We'll examine video art works about children and adolescents here as well as black and LGBTQIA+ issues. Women's issues are given more space in the following chapter. But we start here with men. What makes a man?

MATTHEW BARNEY

Endocrinologists are interested in testosterone and 'maleness'. Medically there really *is* such a thing as 'male toxicity'. Most endocrinologists will have experience of dealing with an angry patient on exogenous testosterone for a deficiency state (e.g. after pituitary surgery) as with the occasional frantic phone call saying some man is smashing up the place – 'he's your patient and he says he's on testosterone!'

Elevated levels of circulating testosterone may be associated with anger outbursts and aggression (Geniole et al., 2020). Depot intramuscular preparations of the hormone may cause unpredictable peaks with subsequent mood issues (Bhasin et al., 2018).

Given the pharmacokinetics of a depot and its prolonged effects, some endocrinologists prefer the use of patches/daily preparations.

Testotoxicosis exists too: this is a rare endocrine condition that can cause precocious puberty in boys. It's an autosomal dominant disorder caused by an activating mutation of the luteinizing hormone (LH) receptor which in turn causes increased testosterone production by Leydig cells in the testes (Nabhan & Eugster, 2019). In adults – again very rarely – an LH producing pituitary tumour can also sometimes cause elevated testosterone production. Of course, a *much* commoner cause of higher-than-normal circulating testosterone is seen following its exogenous use, that is, the aforementioned prescription for men with subnormal testosterone levels or that seen in those who abuse anabolic steroids, often a bodybuilder or an athlete.

American artist Matthew Barney knows a fair bit about athletes and performance; he's an expert too on the cultural implications of male toxicity. His *Cremaster Cycle* (1994–2002) is titled after the muscle responsible for the cremasteric reflex that raises and protects the testes. His *Cremaster* sequence of videos (1–5) lasts a vast 398 minutes. Many sequences are visually stunning and urgently presented but critics have not been slow to accuse the artist of obscurantism. Plot is not Barney's forte: images are. The cycle is said to feature anatomical allusions to the position of the reproductive organs during the embryonic process of sexual differentiation. That's a bit of a leap in my view. My own memory is of a scene from *Cremaster 4* set on the Isle of Man (*gettit?*) where motorbikes with sidecars chase one another on the TT race around the island. What looks like a dissected-out testicle slithers on the chassis of one bike. Yuk.

As for male toxicity itself, Barney ticks off various signifiers: here's a taurine Norman Mailer playing Harry Houdini, over there is the murderer Gary Gilmore; big Cadillacs crash into one another. There are more bulls and satyrs, American football references and Canadian Mounties, a guy in a kilt. We see Finn McCool fighting with Fingal on the Giant's Causeway. The *Cremaster* films are weird but occasionally wonderful. You might see them as a corrective to earlier surrealist works – the worlds of Dalí and Max

Ernst - that were often brutally misogynistic. In Barney's works, we could argue that women are idealized, men demonized. Barney's strange and convoluted worlds ask what might it mean to be man, a *mensch*?

His films are not available on DVD (20 copies were made on disc and sold for hundreds of thousands of dollars) and are only rarely screened – access is thus complicated. This highlights another difference between art video and standard cinema. A trailer and a useful brief critical commentary are, however, available on YouTube and worth a look.

RINEKE DIJKSTRA

Physicians caring for adults try to listen hard to histories from their patients; we study them carefully as they speak. In comparison to paediatric care this process is relatively straightforward as most adults have established their own internal identity and know how to explain themselves both verbally and non-verbally. Children are developing their personality, their identity, and thus history taking – looking for clues – is much more of a challenge. Rineke Dijkstra is an expert in photographic portraiture and has made videos of children that reward study as an insight into the development of character and identity in children. Paediatricians should see her work.

Take *Ruth Drawing Picasso, Tate Liverpool, UK* (2009) for instance. This can be viewed as an exercise in focus, a child here seen concentrating as best as she can on a task. A girl with red hair – aged around nine years – sits on the gallery floor. She's wearing her school uniform – grey jumper, white shirt, red tie and red hairband. She has what looks like bulky Ugg boots on. Her paper is in her lap and we watch her as she looks up at the Picasso off-screen, then down to her pad where we hear her scrawl her copy.

She clamps her mouth tight in concentration, looks over at a pal in competition of a sort; she's socializing. This is all good. This is all *healthy*. We make the kind of judgement that we make every day at the clinic – she's attentive, attending to her task. Neurologically she appears – as discussed earlier – *grossly intact*. Emotionally she seems content, comfortable even. So what holds *our* attention then? Why is this everyday event – a kid drawing at a museum – so compelling?

Two reasons: both applicable to paediatrics. The first is her pose – she appears, in painterly terms, foreshortened. The healthcare worker seeing this might even be reminded of achondroplasia and other forms of dwarfism. Maybe it's the word 'Picasso' in the title that makes the viewer think of the classic Spanish painters, Picasso's dialogue with Velasquez, and in turn Velasquez's *Las Meninas*. There's a sudden burst of pity in the viewer that asks – does little Ruth have restricted growth? No, she does not: she's just normally small ... it's just those Ugg boots that throw you off; they seem to shorten her.

The second feature that hits the emotions on looking at the video is a variant of pity not uncommon to clinical practice: the pity of aspiration. Ruth is doing her very best – we watch her intense concentration but we know this is hard work for her. We know her talent will never, ever, match that of Picasso. And this is another reason we as carers strive to look after kids. They have potential. We don't know what they will end up achieving. So, like Ruth herself, we keep trying to do our best. We have a duty to care for the coming generations ....

Another of Dijkstra's works – *The Weeping Woman* (2009) – is a three-screen piece featuring some of Ruth's schoolmates, boys and girls, all wearing the same school uniform. They are looking at Picasso's painting and occasionally speak to one another and give their interpretation of the artist's very adult (in the sense of emotional) portrait.

Again what we might call the 'Paediatrician Gaze' notes that they are all healthy kids, albeit not obviously privileged; their melodious Scouse accents suggest working class backgrounds. Some gestures are clearly appropriated from their parents or from TV. Boys lean an elbow on another's shoulders. Their own quizzical faces reflect Picasso's intention that we study distress. Their puzzled looks reveal the challenge of interpretation: trying to solve the mystery of an adult's breakdown. As an exercise for the paediatric carer in training you might watch each child in turn and wonder where you think they are in their mental and emotional development. They look as if they are on the right track as they prepare for adulthood. But first, there's adolescence to get through ....

RYAN TRECARTIN

With Trecartin, (born 1981) we move forward developmentally and study the teenage years. Transitional clinics caring for adolescents (too old for paediatric play spaces, too young for adult waiting rooms) are becoming more and more common for many specialties such as diabetes and oncology. Adolescents have their own challenges, their own obsessions and often their own language. They are, too, early adopters of new technology much to the envy and frustration of their parents and carers. As Professor Joe Moran (2023) noted recently 'most of this year's undergraduates were born between September 2003 and August 2004' with 'no memory of a world without broadband'. This is Generation Z.

Ryan Trecartin knows this generation all too well. A Los Angeles-based artist Trecartin has been feted by no less a figure than the late Peter Schjeldahl, the chief art critic of the *New Yorker* for many years. Schjeldahl thought Trecartin 'the most consequential artist to have emerged since the nineteen-eighties'. Why the fuss and what might a view of Trecartin's video works offer those who look after adolescents?

Trecartin's videos give us a privileged insight into the world of today's adolescent minds, bouncing as they do, often manically, between various social media platforms – TikTok, Instagram, etc. – to create hyperactive, soap-opera style dramas that feature much make-up, games with gender fluidity and the forming of identity. The polyphony of voices in Trecartin's work recall listening to a Robert Altman movie – we try to make sense of the overlap cross of conversations. Videos such as *I-Be Area* (2007) that appears to be about cloning and adoption are sometimes incomprehensible, but then the argot of adolescents often is.

Trecartin's generation live in a post-MTV world where what might once have been diagnosed as Attention Deficit/Hyperactivity

Disorder (ADHD) now seems a kind of norm. Adolescents flit from one topic to another with frightening ease; they are energy incarnate, never sitting still. Knights-move thinking is common. And they experiment with adult ideas: in *Junior War* (2013) we see kids getting high, getting drunk, starting fires, speeding in cars, chucking TV sets around – in short kids playing with boundaries. Incoherence is everywhere. Adolescents are not consistent. Trecartin reminds us of this incessantly.

Unsurprisingly his work can be tiring – just as caring for adolescents can be exhausting. As critic Calvin Tomkins (2014) writes: 'The action is propelled by characters making loopy declarative statements about themselves, as young people tend to do, and doing inexplicable things ...'. Trecartin is currently *the* artist reflecting what Tompkins calls 'a place of multiple individual narratives unfolding simultaneously, of shifting identities and genders, of triumphant consumerism, and of young people yakking maniacally into cell phones ...'. That place we call Now.

Massimiliano Gioni is the chief curator of the New Museum, NYC. If someone could be said to be at the cutting edge of the Now and the New it is he. Here he is on Trecartin: 'I felt this was the voice of a different age and a different time, a different sexuality, a different kind of behaviour'.

Trecartin's fast-paced editing and his use of psychedelic colours chimes too with the nuttiness of adolescence. Healthcare workers, like art critics, may find his work baffling but there's no denying the recognition factor when you confront his videos. You think – *I've been there* – both in your own life and when caring for adolescents. Faced with a troubled teenager rejecting the use of insulin, or forgetting to take their asthma medication, or taking an inadvertent/attention-seeking overdose, you think – *cut the kid some slack*. They'll grow out of it.

Much literature on Generation Z has been critical but a recent book – *Gen Z, Explained* (Katz, Ogilvie, Shaw, & Woodhead, 2021) – argues optimistically and convincingly that they are an extraordinarily thoughtful, promising and perceptive group of people. Attention is also drawn to the 'fine-grained' identities of Generation Z with the authors saying 'identities forged in this digital age are intricate mixes of attributes, the result of careful and ongoing discovery'.

ADRIAN PIPER

Adrian Margaret Piper is an American conceptual artist interested in 'otherness' and racism. We should highlight Piper's early video work *Cornered* (1988). Here she begins by saying quite simply: 'I'm black'. Piper explains to those surprised in the audience that she may look fair-skinned and 'pass' for white but she chooses to identify as black. Piper challenges assumptions, notions of superiority. Her work is deliberately uncomfortable and insists on questioning white supremacy. She stresses the genetic reality that many 'white' people have black ancestry. We're reminded powerfully of the Nazi nonsense about eugenics and their pejorative talk about 'mischlings' – people of mixed race. There's a strong argument that Piper's work on racial identity be recommended as essential viewing for medical and nursing students before they even begin working with patients. Her work exposes hidden seams of racism and sexism that corrupt our lives and – by implication – impair our healthcare systems.

ARTHUR JAFA

Arthur Jafa grew up in Mississippi. We might see him as a twenty-first century version of John Heartfield, the Weimar-era Dadaist who used photomontage, collage, to great political effect. Jafa's *Love is the Message, The Message is Death* (2016) is an effecting and effective collage of video moments – in his words 'self-owned documentation' – that highlights the triumphs and traumas of Black America to the soundtrack of Kanye West's *Ultralight Beam*. We see heroes and heroines like Muhammed Ali and Miles Davis, Coretta King and Nina Simone, spliced with appalling incidents of racial violence, racial injustice. The KKK and armed police are seen brutalizing the innocent. The work says to white healthcare workers – here is evidence of black success, our worth, but here too is what your people have done to us, remember this when you are charged with our welfare.

Jafa pulls striking images from the Internet– what he calls 'a tidal wave of documentation', that watery metaphor we began this book with – with intent to deliberately disturb. He juxtaposes wealth with poverty, success with failure. He asks us to look without flinching – see this for what it is – an imperative for carers. Again we're asked to look at complicated things with *distance*. In a video interview for the Louisiana Channel he stresses the importance of such distance – a detachment that carers must develop too. He says he tries to be 'super-clinical, almost forensic at things we're looking at'. Like a clinician, he stresses that he needs to see the problem clearly but at the same time knows he has to 'flip the switch' and be *inside* and *outside* the issue: 'Be both in and out of it at the same time'. We can see this as another insight into empathy with the sick.

SIN WAI KIN

Given the over-exaggerated fears from certain reactionary commentators regarding trans rights and trans issues, it's refreshing to find the exhilarating work of Sin Wai Kin. Kin creates characters in their videos that undermine binary sexual narratives – as such their work is educative viewing for those who care for trans individuals, which means *everyone* in the caring professions. If you don't want to care for people, care without prejudice, find another job. Kin's characters are larger than life in appearance, reminiscent of sci-fi figures, or manga comic book stars. Kin's world is fantastical and in constant flux. Their work challenges standard tropes of feminine and masculine 'ideal' imagery, that Kin suggests we've been 'conditioned to want'. Kin affirms that 'we all have an experience of existing in binary narratives': this is correct even for the majority 'normals' who sit comfortably in their gender identity.

All doctors and nurses need to have the empathic imaginative capacity to understand the issues that face patients with other gender identities. Think not? Ask yourself if you've ever read a book where the narrator is not of your gender. Have you *never* sympathized with a character not of your gender in a play, in a film, on a TV programme? Have you never thought that you don't fit into a category, be it one deemed to be political, national, racial, sexual? If not maybe you shouldn't be looking after people. The current popularity of drag artists on TV and the ongoing empowerment of trans people would suggest Kin's Taoist-informed work questioning all sorts of binaries will have continued relevance to carers for some time to come.

GILLIAN WEARING

Wearing, given her interest in masks and identity, has also made works dealing with gender issues. Wearing has disguised herself as a man (including members of her own family) for carefully manipulated photographs. She has also posed as Claude Cahun, an artist from the 1920s. Cahun was seriously ahead of the curve in her own 'gender-fluid' self-portraits. Wearing's works have an eerie charge and remind us, as with Adrian Piper's work on race, of her (and our) genetic inheritance. We *do* look like our uncles, our aunts, our cousins. Those clichés we utter when faced with a new baby – *he's got his mother's nose/she's got his father's ears* – are all true.

TIKTOK 6

Where to start? We're talking millions of posted videos about identity. Arguably the use of social media to comment on identity issues has been the defining characteristic of our time. Some see this – the so-called 'woke' generation – as empowering: others as threatening to the hegemony of Goffman's (1963) 'normals'. For Generation Z revealing weakness and talking about stigma is 'honest, authentic and appreciated' (Katz et al., 2021). They cite – to use another medical example – the popularity of the Canadian model Winnie Harlow, who 'celebrates rather than hides her vitiligo'.

In terms of medical care, there are many quite brilliant streams made by individuals 'labelled' with illnesses – diabetes, epilepsy, infertility and so on. These are people who argue that they are *not* to be reduced or traduced in identity, to become a mere diagnostic 'label', to be considered as mere statistics in public health records. There's a very strong case to be made that some of these videos be incorporated into medical teaching on such illnesses – the people who have made these non-arty video self-portraits are telling us what it is *really* like to live with the condition and how these may impact on the day-to-day issues of life. This is an incredible resource with a ridiculous ease of access that should be used in these times where education is hard-pressed given clinical demands and governmental cutbacks. Such videos arguably make for ideal self-directed learning.

7

WOMEN

Video art has played a not inconsiderable role in the emancipation of women since the 1960s. This chapter will review key works and also suggest where these can be used in both teaching healthcare workers and also where they may be of use in potential clinical scenarios. Video art has been indisputably more challenging and confrontational than mainstream cinema when it comes to feminist issues.

PIPILOTTI RIST

Women workers get a raw deal in the medical world: several specialties – orthopaedics notoriously – still have a marked gender imbalance. Pay discrepancy is still, unbelievably, a real live issue and senior positions are, persistently, overwhelmingly, male. Female doctors are mistaken for nurses on a daily basis. Nurses and doctors are at the receiving end of unwelcome sexual overtures and violence from male patients. How to empower women in medicine is an ongoing project but meanwhile video art can point towards a better, fairer, world. If asked to choose one work that might embolden activists, one that might encourage women in medicine to keep up the pressure, to insist on parity, I'd choose *Ever Is Over All* (1997) by Pipilotti Rist.

We see two screens and on the leftward we watch, in slow motion, a young woman in a blue dress stride down a street.

She's wearing red shoes, high heels, like Dorothy from the Wizard of Oz. She's got something in her hands; something orange that appears on the right screen, something floral; there's what looks like petals. The soundtrack is a woman's voice humming lazily. Here we see (what appears to be) a calm world. A xylophone trill accompanies the voice. There's a cut and we now see her face on, she's beaming, she looks ecstatic. There are cars parked at the side of the road, vehicles innocent of what's about to happen to them. That object in her hand is now raised – it seems to have a green stalk and it's about the size of a child's golf putter. A man passing her looks worried. With a twirl of her body she crashes the object into a passenger window of one of the parked cars and smashes the glass with glee. Boom! The soundtrack is interrupted by the amplified smack of breaking glass. We recognize that the flower she's holding isn't a real Red Hot Poker plant but a metallic fake. A weapon ....

She strides on and we make out a figure walking behind her – a policewoman in full uniform. She's in trouble now – or is she? The flower weapon is raised again and – *crack* – she's gone and smashed another car window! She's nonchalant, grinning again at her transgression. The policewoman passes her, is in no rush to rebuke her, and indeed gives her an admiring salute. A man passes by and looks on, incredulous. This is a world Not Ruled By Men. A third car window gets demolished. A kid on a bike and an old woman pass by, indifferent to the carnage. It's the men who look scared ....

How to make sense of *Ever Is Over All*? Is it a feminist revenge fantasy? That's one way of reading it. As Peggy Phelan et al. (2001) writes:

> The phallic flower is wielded by a woman in a conservative dress; her counterpart, the police woman officer wearing the clothes of the state and representing 'the law of the father' applauds the power of the phallic woman.

The bucolic scenes in the adjoining screen might be read as a reminder of feminine grace and the benign impact of Mother Nature. But don't be fooled ....

For most of my working career, there was a distinct minority of women sat around high-pressured hospital committee boards, regional and national bodies; you saw women surrounded by men. Institutional misogyny is still problematic; some men need to change and challenge this issue. It's good to think that *Ever Is Over All* could inspire women if they ever sense bullying by the majority.

Rist plays around with the video form in works that clearly reference pop music videos – as such she can be considered an exemplar of the artist unafraid to use cutting-edge technology – what the *New Yorker* critic Peter Schjeldahl calls 'the universal cyberair'. Rist is interested in the body – she's called the eyes 'blood-operated cameras'. She made *Bloodclip* (1993), a two-minute video ode to menstruation. In explanation she said:

> *I would be happy if young girls who have their first period see it as an occasion for loud rejoicing. Bring the blood out into the open, show this red fluid, this wonderful sap.*

Again she refers to botanical allusions.

Bloodclip begins with a scanning shot that sees Rist's face as she lies on the ground. Her body is dotted with sparkling gems. As the camera reaches her crotch the number of gems increases, obscuring her vulva. There's then a cut to the clothed Rist who removes her white pants to show a bright red bloodstain. In the background a female pop singer is singing *yeah, yeah*, to an exuberant tune. A saxophone blares as the camera scans down a pale leg with a long line of blood. More streaks dribble down as the singer goes on. This could look grotesque but there is an undoubted sense of celebration, of joy. We're reminded of Paul McCarthy and his ketchup. Or is this the gooey raspberry sauce we once had dripped over our ice creams at the beach? No – this is *real* blood.

A globe appears implying that this event is a universal affair for most women. Rist is attempting what seems impossible – taking the outrageous haemorrhagic effusions of the Viennese Actionists and taming them, feminizing them. She's trying to demystify blood and menstruation, trying to remove its stigma, its association with trauma. How young women perceive the menarche is Rist's real concern here. If she reassures just one young girl she's done her job.

On a personal level another work – *Sip My Ocean* (1996) – has strong anxiolytic properties that might benefit the over-worried. This piece might be the definitional 'immersive' work, an admittedly overused term in video/art criticism. The footage is shot underwater and the blues seen on the twin screens are hypnotic, near hallucinogenic. We float visually along the seafloor, glimpse bodies and disembodied eyes. In short, we relax. I'd recommend this work to the psychological support teams that are now routinely available to those working in oncology services. The work actively de-stresses the viewer. This is Rist's chill-out zone.

YOKO ONO

Undressing when you're at the clinic: this is a source of potential embarrassment, a situation where patients generally feel extremely vulnerable, even with a chaperone present. *Cut Piece* (1964) by Yoko Ono highlights the vulnerability of women and yet Ono herself (perhaps predictably given her reputation for being contrarian) has been more ambiguous in discussion about the meaning of the work. She sits on a stage, impassive to the people who come up to her with a pair of scissors; men and women snip away at her clothes. Ono's lack of interaction, her absence of agency, is the real point here. This is what it feels like to be examined, to be merely a body, an unthinking thing. That the audience participates at all tells us something about crowds and power, how the body can be reified, turned into a mere commodity, a thing. There's one section that makes for distinctly uncomfortable viewing where one man cuts and cuts away at her blouse. There's the anxiety that this is a preliminary action before a more disturbing form of assault.

Did Ono need to remind us of our barbarian nature after the obvious atrocities of the Second World War, the Holocaust and Hiroshima? Yes, because we forget. Or aren't taught. As said it's not unreasonable to remind medical students of the Holocaust and its lessons. History is slippery and not always well explained at school. Two medical students in my clinic – circa 2016 – did not know who Joseph Stalin was. Use of Ono's *Cut Piece* might facilitate debate among medical students as to the representation of aggression and violence towards women and what the caring professions might do to ameliorate this blight.

ANA MENDIETA

If Yoko Ono's work challenges men and empowers women then the Cuban-American artist Ana Mendieta took such strategies to another level. She made several films that examine violence against women. Again her story should be of major interest to anyone in health care systems charged with looking after women, that is, us all. Her silent video *Sweating Blood* (1973) is exactly that – we stare at her, face on, as trickles of blood dribble down her face. The work was in response to the murder of an American student, Sarah Ann Ottens.

Mendieta's own subsequent death following a fall from a skyscraper in 1985 – did she jump or was she pushed? – remains highly controversial. Even in a world as highly publicized, as *visible* as that of contemporary art the cause of Mendieta's death is still unsolved. Her artist husband – Carl Andre – was acquitted of her murder but key questions remain: in the eyes of many women in the art world men are still a big problem. The medical world knows this too.

TRACEY EMIN

We begin with Super 8 footage of the seaside at Margate and then see a wall with the title in caps: *Why I Never Became a Dancer*. This 1995 video by Tracey Emin is typically autobiographical and sketches Emin's youth and private life. The video is brutally honest and tells us how she left school at 13 years because she hated it. She hangs around cafes and drinks cider on the beach.

> And then there was sex. It was something you could just do. And it was free.

Emin then talks of how it didn't matter – to the men – that she was underage. Her sad voiceover accompanies images of feral seagulls squawking, sordid alleyways, sleazy amusement arcades and fish 'n' chip shops. Escape from abuse comes in the form of dancing, the dance floor, where she feels free. Dreams of contests and making the finals in London. A gang of men calls her 'slag' and shouts the word in repeat. She leaves the town she grew up in and names her abusers. Cut to her jiving again and smiling again – for Emin revenge is sweet, her success mocks her abusers.

This work gives an acute insight into the challenges and pressures that face young working-class women. Emin is acute and frank about her early, often abusive, experiences with sex and men. Again we can argue that this should be mandatory viewing for those tasked (psychiatrists/nurses/A+E staff/GUM clinics) with looking after at-risk women, the undereducated, the exploited.

We should also draw attention to Emin's later experiences with an aggressive pelvic cancer requiring radical surgery as evidenced in a TV interview cited in the references. Those involved in oncological services will find her experiences as a patient worthy of examination and discussion.

8

NEW TECHNOLOGIES/
NEW VISIONS

There's a date stamp on this chapter and on this book, let's be optimistic: *Best Before 2033*. It won't take long for many of the so-called innovations mentioned here to become outdated. Any survey of new developments will appear outmoded in time. Having said that I'd like to highlight the work of a few artists practicing right now whose ideas should survive, whose videos have received steady praise and who seem likely to attain, if not canonical status, a lengthy period of relevance.

ED ATKINS

Ed Atkins uses cutting-edge CGI effects to make video works that destabilize the viewer and render the familiar strange. He's fascinated by death, as we detailed earlier with his curating of Stan Brakhage's work on autopsies. Atkins' own videos are sometimes melancholic but are clearly insightful into clinical depression as with *Ribbons* (2014). Here we encounter a strikingly convincing CGI animation, an avatar of a sad young man drinking beer and smoking: he's harming himself and he's lonely – we hear his mournful singing of Randy Newman's 'I Think It's Going to Rain Today'. We see his line of drained pint glasses, his empty cigarette packets, and his rubbishy tattoos. He says 'help me communicate without debasement, darling' to the accompaniment of Newman's plaintive piano notes. His facial gestures look hauntingly real and yet we know they are fake, not the real thing, they're only based on the reality. Our sense – as viewers – of his de-realization and estrangement gives an acute insight into the symptomatology of those who have *actual* clinical depression.

Speaking of 'fake' we are now living in a time of 'deep fakes', video and computer technology that can render the unreal in a hyperreal fashion. This can be viewed as a troubling political development – a tool to create untruths. How deep fakes might impact on healthcare has yet to be determined but the efforts of the anti-vaccine community during the COVID-19 pandemic does not encourage optimism. There are already fears that scientific publications could be threatened by image fabrication (Wang, Zhou, Yang, & Yu, 2022). On the other hand, Generation Z and the younger Generation Alpha are savvy and on to the fakers. Time will tell ....

CHRISTIAN MARCLAY

There's never enough time in medicine. Time is stressful. Sometimes working in medicine feels you're a bit like the silent movie come-dian Harold Lloyd hanging from a clock high above the street and the void below. Disaster beckons for the dangling man. Carers in the medical profession work long hours. Friendships and family relationships suffer. Talk to doctors about time and they'll tell you of shifts where they've had to see ten patients in an hour with eight waiting to be seen. And the rest ....

Doctors are clerking in with one eye on the clock before hav-ing to leave for the morning ward round. My guess is that every carer thinks about time and the *actual* time at some point during a consultation. Strategies to get patients out of a room like standing up or guiding them by the elbow to the door, are well known. The only time when time is not the enemy is in the private sector. Time there is money. It's not hard to imagine the more venal members of the healthcare professions saying to themselves: *Keep them talking. Keep ordering tests. Ker-ching!*

Time is one of Christian Marclay's subjects. He says he 'doesn't have much time' because 'time is precious'. There's much to learn and admire about how Marclay sees time operating. *The Clock* (2010) is something of a masterpiece, a 24-hour work, a 24-hour timepiece in itself, which few have seen in its entirety. The work can be considered an exemplar as regards our earlier discussions around dipping in and out of a work; time flows. *The Clock* uses stunning cutting and sampling techniques to create a video made from over 12,000 movie clips. The video works both as art *and* as a clock itself because it begins with images of clocks and watches that indicate the *precise* time in the real world.

What exactly do we encounter in *The Clock*? Let's take a section beginning around five past twelve in the afternoon. This starts with someone reading the BBC news then cuts to a clock telling us the time, our own time. We watch the red second hand sweep round. The next sequence has a bedside clock sat beside a mirror with a white streak of cocaine. A man traces his finger in the powder and then rubs his gums. We watch him select his clothes from his dresser and sing a song; we recognize Richard Gere from Paul Schrader's movie *American Gigolo*. Yet another cut focusses on another clock, this time with Arabic numerals. Then we see a monochrome be-suited John Steed from *The Avengers* armed with brolly and bowler. Marclay uses video *and* TV clips in addition to movie samples.

Steed finds a dead body. As with being on-call we remember being paged, our attention diverted elsewhere, to come and confirm someone has died (*now please!*) only to be interrupted yet again as we confront the corpse, asked by another to hurry up and see someone else, someone still alive. *The Clock* is about *interruption*: our working day flows like the video, time moves on, but we are endlessly pestered to do something else. Attention is constantly being requested elsewhere. Medicine is all about interruption.

'You wouldn't have the time, Miss?' says a voice. Doctors and nurses get asked this *many* times in a day. *I know you're a busy man, but can I just ask* ... Even the shift in genres we witness in *The Clock* – from Horror to Western (blue-eyed Henry Fonda has just appeared on screen looking fearful) – mimics a day on-call.

One minute we are asked about a life-threatening cardiology issue, another a minor orthopaedic complaint. Next up in *The Clock* we see a character getting fired, maybe for poor timekeeping; carers recognize this threat all too well. Every doctor and nurse worries about timekeeping and keeping their job.

Then there's the humour of time itself: alarms going off in the middle of lectures. We see Laurel and Hardy dealing with a clock going barmy. We're reminded of people who set their watches a permanent five minutes ahead – *just in case*. Watching *The Clock* we recognize old faces, old actors, this again like an on-call shift where we see repeat attenders, and our memories get to work. *The Clock*, with its startling moments of recognition – *I've seen this before!* – chimes with making a diagnosis. Pattern recognition is key to clinical success. Artists and carers are both attuned to patterns.

And now here's Crocodile Dundee on the screen; he can tell the time by looking up at the sun. Many care workers on shifts get skilled at clues to the time from the amount of outside light. Dawn is breaking and that ward round beckons. An excerpt from *Mission Impossible* reminds us we can't always get things done on time. Sometimes it really *is* time to get help.

In an interview Marclay says he thinks we are much happier when we don't think about time. He goes on to say his video is really about 'the present': again this is another insight relevant to carers given that being on-call can seem like a permanent present. There's a paradox here because the clips in Marclay's work are all from the past, past movies watched in the here and now, some of them referenced in Schlozman's *Film*. But there's another parallel with being on-call given that dealing with different cases in the present (as a busy GP or hospital doctor or nurse) is still to be confronted by the past, lessons learned, the persistent question-ing: *where have I seen this before?* What did I do when I saw this situation last? Didn't I read something about this condition not so long ago?

The Clock is also a study of anxiety and boredom and death, death as *memento mori* – as Marclay says of the work: 'you're con-stantly reminded of death'. And this too is absolutely the case as a healthcare worker. Like an on-call shift, there are moments in *The Clock* where time goes by very fast, usually in action sequences that recall times when we're engaged in some emergency. The happy flipside of being busy, as we all know, is that time goes by quickly; the shift comes to end before we know it. The corollary, as with *The Clock*, is that some sections are boring, not much happens, and time is drawn out, stretched like a piece of chewing gum. Again, all carers will recognize these moments – nothing is happening and it's 3.00 a.m. There's five hours to go before time for home. Time flies, time crawls.

The Clock has a deeply hypnotic effect; its viewing may even be of value in certain clinical situations. We might argue it gives an insight into attention deficit hyperactivity disorder (ADHD) given the rapidity of Marclay's cuts. This is how we might imagine those afflicted with *real* ADHD live as they try to interact with the world. *The Clock*, as critic Andrew Graham-Dixon says 'worries away obsessively' again and again – just like those on a busy shift on an acute medical unit. There's an all-pervading sense of anxiety watching *The Clock* that's extremely reminiscent of being on-call.

JORDAN WOLFSON

The history of art is layered with images that try to capture and understand suffering. One thinks of Edvard Munch's cachectic victims in the sick room. The condition depicted, tuberculosis, was not being addressed – the bacterium itself was not the subject – the patient was. The late twentieth century saw an urgency to deal with a deadly new infective threat – HIV – that directly influenced the often-polemical nature of art produced by the likes of General Idea, Group Material, and Félix González-Torres. As a consequence, there exists – I suspect – more works of art about HIV and AIDS than any other illness. But again, as with Munch, the artistic focus was on the raw social impact of the disease rather than the virus itself. The pathogen was not the star of the show – perhaps that had to wait until artists were relieved to know that control of the disease was in sight, that the existential threat of the virus might soon be held in check. Enter the art-world's current *enfant terrible*: Jordan Wolfson.

How can we be sure that a new artist is worthy of attention, that their work has become 'iconic'? The classic critical trajectory was via the apparatus of print media. Decades after the (often shocking) debut appearance of an artwork, a consensus was generally arrived at in the art press and the (previously appalled) public would then queue in their droves to catch a glimpse of the once-forbidden treasure. Think of Manet's *Olympia* or Duchamp's *Nude Descending a Staircase, No. 2* (1912). But with the advent of modern media and video this process has become significantly accelerated. We can look at the hit numbers of YouTube viewing. And by doing so we can reach the rapid conclusion that Jordan Wolfson's images have gone viral in more ways than one. He has been welcomed to the hall of greats, mentioned in the same breath as (gulp) Picasso, Warhol and Jeff Koons before he has even reached the age of 40 years. Whether this acclaim will be sustained is unclear.

When I last checked the online excerpts from his recent show at David Zwirner's gallery in New York City (which closed on 19 April 2022) they had been seen by over one million viewers. Why? In short because his work is a new way of looking at the body and its vulnerability, about what we see and how we look at other people. And viruses ....

Wolfson's *Raspberry Poseur* (2012) is a digital video that lasts nearly fourteen minutes. The use of CGI gives the work an immediate contemporary impact – you have seen this sort of manipulation watching movies for kids. But those talented folks at Pixar have little of Wolfson's daring; this is work for adults. He conjures up a balletic condom twisting languidly in the air. As it flies past trendy interiors we see it spill its contents: scarlet love-hearts. And then? Enter the virus. Bouncy, bright crimson retroviruses boing up and down on their elastic projecting glycoproteins over images of relaxed young Americans at play. Wolfson's point here, I suspect, is the indifference of the virus. We might seem content in our plastic materialistic world but the virus is too. That's what parasites do, hide in plain sight amongst us. The clinician is reminded that we must look for HIV when we may not initially suspect it – in the elderly (who *do* have sex and some take heroin too!), in all those tame admissions labelled wrongly as 'chest infection', or 'gastro-enteritis' or 'viral meningitis'. These may be the presentational symptoms of HIV infection.

The highlight, so far, of Wolfson's meteoric career is the sculpture *Female Figure* (2013) that can be viewed on video online. This is an animatronic dancer who gyrates somewhat in the manner of a manipulated pop figure like Miley Cyrus. She wears a frightening witch mask and is umbilically connected by a metal rod to a mirror. Via the wonders of expensive visual recognition software her eyes can follow you, the viewer, around the room. This is a neat joke on that old cliché about great portraiture. The effect is eerily disturbing and quite clearly a jibe at the tawdry excesses of the male gaze. This work takes sculpture of the body and its representation to a new level of verisimilitude; we are a long way from Degas' *Little Dancer* and now truly in the uncanny, disturbing world of a Sci-Fi Geppetto.

Wolfson's appropriated photograph *Helen Keller* (2007) is, I think, a key to his greater concerns – the struggle to communicate as exemplified by the famous deaf and blind author. Wolfson's works hint that (despite the profusion of information engendered by the Internet) there are still grave difficulties in saying what we want to say, to capture what we mean, when we are faced with gross insensitivities, or when we're in pain. Wolfson trains his discomfiting gaze at our venal Wall Street world of psychotic acquisitiveness and degraded notions of caring. Some critics imply that he may merely be washing his hands, like Pontius Pilate, of any personal responsibility for this mess. Others argue his work revels in projecting and exposing the fake masks we wear, as with Gillian Wearing. Masks that obscure and prevent us from saying – *Ecce Homo* – behold the man.

But Wolfson embraces, indeed loves, controversy; his most notorious work is called *Real Violence* (2017). The viewer uses virtual reality glasses (age restriction 17 years or over with trigger warning supplied) to watch a two-minute iPhone video (Jeffries, S. 2018). We're in Manhattan on a lovely day and see a young man kneeling on the sidewalk. We then watch Wolfson smash a baseball bat into the guy's skull. Wolfson stomps on his head. There's blood: real or McCarthy-like ketchup? Or is it a virtual deepfake, more CGI trickery? Life goes on as normal elsewhere. People walk by. What we see looks sickeningly real. But it isn't – the 'victim' is another animatronic creation – what we're watching is an upmarket update, a high-tech upgrade, of a Tom and Jerry cartoon.

When asked if he's a moralist Wolfson replied 'I hope not' – but he's being disingenuous. His work clearly references the traumatic and its effects on the body. Artists have an allergy to being labelled as 'moralists' – witness the differing silences of Marcel Duchamp (acting clever) and Andy Warhol (acting dumb). Or Nabokov's strictures when the label was applied to him – artists think the term 'moralist' restricts them and many would rather they were viewed as mirrors to society, mere storytellers rather than righteous preachers. But it's undeniable that Wolfson is addressing the human propensity to violence, particularly anti-Semitic violence: witness the soundtrack to *Real Violence* where a man in the background sings Hanukkah blessings (Schwartz, 2017). Is this Wolfson's Jewish revenge fantasy for the Holocaust? As with Schlozman's arguments about psychosis in *Film* we see a video dealing with a highly charged subject. There's a Tarantino-like feel to Wolfson's *Real Violence*: an attempt to understand explosive rage.

You can watch the public's reactions to *Real Violence* on YouTube – some of the youngsters watching it rip their headsets off, appalled. Others laugh, maybe in on the gag that it's all virtual, maybe because they themselves are undiagnosed psychopaths. But Wolfson is showing us that the fake isn't real: that its actual *reality* we should truly fear. His is the world of gaming too – an enormous constituency that healthcare workers need to understand. The gaming arena can be disturbing – those deep fakes again – but it shouldn't be ignored.

VIDEO GAMING: CAN VIDEO CAUSE HARM?

A recent review has highlighted the health effects of too much gaming (Grinspoon, 2022). There are the known physical complaints: relatively minor issues such as repetitive stress injuries – carpal tunnel syndrome, "gamer's thumb" – and others that are potentially much more significant such as obesity.

Psychologically, some may become addicted to gaming videos. Whether this is a unique syndrome or not is open to question but the American Psychological Association has identified nine criteria that may be help define the problem. One paper suggests that up to 1 per cent of Americans may have an Internet gaming disorder (Przybylski, Weinstein, & Murayama, 2017). Sleep deprivation has been associated with the 'condition' but clearly further study is needed on the impact of these popular pursuits. Grinspoon recommends the 20-20-20 rule: every 20 minutes try to look at something 20 feet away for 20 seconds. The evidence of benefit after doing this is unclear.

Grinspoon talks too of the mixed results around the putative benefits of gaming, that is, cognitive gains and improved spatial reasoning. Video games may help train people with neurodegenerative disease to improve balance and even contribute to training surgeons on technically difficult operations.

LU YANG

The majority of newly qualified doctors and nurses, support workers and carers, were born in the twenty-first century – Generation Z. Theirs is a digital world with occasional analogue throwbacks. The movies they watch are highly technical affairs involving innovations in computer graphics: many are gamers, and many are indifferent to more traditional modes of entertainment such as theatre or books. They consult social media platforms hundreds of times per day; they are conscious of virtual worlds and create their own avatars. Video appeals to a younger generation precisely because of its newness and its relevance to their lives.

Is it possible to make a video work for this new generation that references manga animation, superheroes, anatomy and feminism – a video that is both educational for those in medical training *and* turns out to be highly amusing? That would be a 'yes'. Lu Yang – a Shanghai-based artist working at the coalface of cutting technologies – has pulled off this trick with *Uterus Man* (2013).

Hers is a highly imaginative digital world that embraces 3D animated technology to examine topics such as neuroscience and gender-fluid sexuality.

Uterus Man begins like a manga cartoon with its rapid gabber/techno beats, its multilingual titles with multiple characters using the Latin alphabet, the Japanese kanji, the Chinese Han; we see the face of the titular hero/heroine. Yang then fast cuts to animations of the human skeleton focussing on the pelvis. There are flashes of text that mention the word 'gene'. Are we to assume that Uterus Man is a genetically modified human – a man who looks like a uterus? We see his arms are the fallopian tubes, his hands the fimbria. He rides a pelvis shaped flying vehicle through tunnels. The word 'DNA' flashes and we see Uterus Man zapping in a circle around animations of the double helix. The face of Uterus Man will be familiar to those into manga comics – he/she is gender fluid, their features are soft, their eyes are huge, hair is pansexual in design. There are more shots of the roving ilium vehicle that looks like something out of H.R. Geiger's dreams, a skeletal beach buggy bouncing over some dunes on the moon.

Now comes the anatomy lesson. Texts appear and disappear in rapid succession illustrating the speed with which young people can interpret visual imagery. Moving down the arms of the fallopian tubes, we see *actual* footage of ovaries taken from both laparoscopic and ultrasonic captures. Uterus Man's chest wall is the uterine cavity itself. Freeze frame on YouTube and you can read: 'the cavity of the body of the uterus is a mere slit flattened antero-posteriorly. It is triangular in shape, the base being formed ...' and so on. Rarely has anatomical education been so much fun.

The pudendal region is of course the cervix and vagina themselves. Again we read texts in both English and Mandarin: the figure spins rapidly on its axis as if it were a parody of old-style TV animations on biology. The techno soundtrack pulses on with Kraftwerk-style vocoder interjections that talk of 'blood energy'. A jet of blood then emerges from Uterus Man's feet as he/she/they power along into deep space; a deliberately humorous feminist reference to menstruation. We remember Pipilotti Rist's earlier TV video. The voice talks of 'blood energy altitude flying'.

The joking intensifies with the next sequence that highlights another of Uterus Man's methods of transportation – the sanitary pad skateboard – this looks exactly like you'd think it would. As with the Silver Surfer, Uterus Man bends his knees and jumps on the board then powers through a neon-lit futurama landscape done in high graphic design.

Uterus Man also uses menstrual blood as weapon like the Marvel comic book character Human Torch attacking with his signature burst of fire: *Flame On!* Then there's something called the 'XY Chromosome Attack' where Uterus Man fires ovum at Y shapes: another laugh-out loud moment. Again all the rapid-fire digital animation is cut with actual shots taken from gynaecological investigations that include MRI scan imagery.

If this anatomical lesson wasn't detailed enough we then get more on the 'pelvis chariot' and a quick primer on bone with its cortical and trabecular aspects labelled. The pelvis chariot can walk and fly and has a hilarious 'deep throat laser cannon', a skull appendage that can fire atomic missiles, again all this intercut with radiological input.

The laughs intensify with a section called 'Summoning the Baby Weapon'. Again we get some real footage of spermatozoa fertilizing an egg intercut with Uterus Man swelling up in pregnancy then delivering a baby and placenta out of his/her feet. The baby can be programmed into 'beast mode' where it yells and stomps like a feral dog. Baby Weapon is Uterus Man's *true* secret capability and we see it swung around on its placenta like a mace. Lu Yang pushes the limits of good taste here but the baby is heard giggling away, clearly enjoying its crazy powers. The umbilical cord is transformed into a whip and the placenta used as a force-field shield against shots of multiplying bacteria.

One of Lu Yang's most recent works – *DOKU the Self* (2022) – transforms her own body and facial features into a gender-neutral avatar. Individuals whose identities are also fluid people her speculative worlds; hers is a future where the digital world is as 'real' as the 'real world', a world of cyborgs in states of permanent change. There is a Buddhist-like questioning here of dualistic thinking on the self, that things are either – as with the texts accompanying the exhibition – natural or artificial, male or female, me or you.

There's the suggestion that the gamer world, the Generation Alpha world of the twenty-first century, the new world of healthcare, may involve a lot more non-dualistic thinking, a new approach to try and free ourselves of ego. Lang's imaginary is one of hope in the face of culture wars and climate disaster.

At the end of *DOKU the Self* Lu Yang's most recent transformation rises into space then shatters into diamond-like splinters, and this time it's the anatomy of her brain that is detailed in all its amazing complexity; yet another novel lesson in neurology and neurosurgery for medics in training, and for Yang yet another allusion to the illusion of the self.

MERIEM BENNANI

A dancing stethoscope? Yes indeed … the rubber earplugs are a pair of jiving feet, the flexible tubing is the body, the bell is the face, the diaphragm is the back of the head. The reference to Disney's *Fantasia* is obvious: we remember Mickey Mouse and those anthropomorphic buckets and brooms. This is a scene from Meriem Bennani's video *Guided Tour of a Spill (CAPS Interlude)* (2021). We're about seven minutes into the sixteen-minute video. A gang of young men is seen flexing their muscles (in anticipation of a fight perhaps) and then suddenly the animated stethoscope snakes up the screen and its dance begins. To a soundtrack of thumping Arabic techno the stethoscope boogies away along with some flying toasters. That's right, toasters … as in those doughty stalwarts of a night on-call, those dysfunctional beasts that (inevitably, regularly) set off multiple hospital alarm systems. The toasters also dance in military formation then the stethoscopes multiply and auscultate the slices of toast, the pop-up mechanism, the grill itself. The bell begins to sing a soul tune. It's all delightfully daft and thrilling.

Bennani is a young Moroccan-born artist based in New York who made number 96 in ArtReview magazine's Power 100 of 2021. Her ideas are on point as regards immigration and freedom of movement – she has invented an imagined world in this video where people can teleport *a la* Star Trek. But those trying to get

into America are held in a detention centre. Like many young artists Bennani is inspired by YouTube videos, in her case from her
own home country. She debuts some of her work on Instagram –
again a common practice for developing artists. Bennani came to
prominence after making a COVID-19 lockdown video of a ghost
town Manhattan called *2 Lizards* (2020). As with Jordan Wolfson
we are on a CGI modified planet only this time one that's less por-
tentous, one that has more humour and less violence. Bennani's
sampling, her zappy productions, have been described by critic
Cat Kron (2021) as a 'YouTube soup' … a 'mashup of hand-held
amateur video and the animated style of 2010s-era electronica
music-videos'.

NAN GOLDIN

We conclude this brief survey of The New with Nan Goldin – the
doyen of late twentieth century New York photography – and
argue that she's still an innovator. How so? By using an old-style
slideshow captured as video? What's so innovative about that? No,
it's her political engagement that interests us here rather than her
use of the form.

Goldin was born in 1953 and has recently influenced the medical
professions in a quite unprecedented manner. Her early work *The
Ballad of Sexual Dependency* (1986) took its title from a Bertolt
Brecht lyric: this was an unflinching pictorial autobiography that
(notoriously) features images from the hard drug subculture of
New York, the addicts and prostitutes, the beaten. One shocking
picture shows Goldin herself bruised after physical abuse from a
boyfriend. Her work predated similar confessional trends in art
as with Tracey Emin and Gillian Wearing. Sean O'Hagan (2014),
writing in the *Guardian*, argued:

> *we are now living to a degree in a world Nan Goldin
> created long before the digital camera and Instagram
> made it ubiquitous: a self-absorbed, often revelatory
> world where the everyday and the exotic exist in uneasy
> cohabitation.*

But although her early works have relevance to healthcare professionals in that they deal with the horror of drug addiction (and Goldin has admitted to a romanticized view of drug misuse at a young age) it's her *current* political stance that has changed the healthcare professions. Despite her past history of heroin addiction a doctor started Goldin on OxyContin for tendonitis; she became quickly addicted to the drug. She went into a rehab facility and learned more about OxyContin and how it was responsible for over 200,000 deaths; how it was marketed; how doctors bought into the lie promoted by the pharmaceutical company that this new synthetic form of opiate was 'harmless', was 'safe'.

Goldin took on the Sackler family responsible for the marketing of the drug. The family made billions from Purdue Pharma, the company that marketed OxyContin. Prior to the scandal the Sackler's were perceived as major philanthropists – in particular as the art world was concerned. If you've been in a major museum/gallery its highly likely you've been in one of the wings they've funded; there are many institutions named after them. As Joanna Walters (2018) reported: 'It (OxyContin) was aggressively marketed to doctors – many of whom were on lavish junkets, given misleading information and paid to give talks on the drug …'

The *New Yorker* columnist Patrick Radden Keefe exposed the family in his forensic dissection of malfeasance, 'Empire of Pain'. Allen Frances, former chair of psychiatry at Duke University is quoted as saying:

> *Their name (Sackler) has been pushed forward as the epitome of good works … but when it comes down to it, they've earned this fortune at the expense of millions of people who are addicted. It's shocking how they have gotten away with it.*

Except now they haven't. Thanks to the efforts of Goldin and others the family has had to pay billions in compensation and specifically $4.5 billion to fund addiction treatment. Various blue-chip-art establishments have distanced themselves from the family.

Goldin's relentless agitation against the use of the drug – the company that produce it, the doctors that promoted and prescribed it – is an important new lesson to the healthcare professions from the world of video art: we must listen to video artists. Indeed Goldin, and her supporters, may arguably have saved more lives than many doctors. Her exposure of greedy unethical 'professionals' shows there's another crucial side to video art and its influence: its practitioners can work as a major corrective to collective delusion, to collective greed.

9

CONCLUSIONS

This has been a personal selection of video recommendations, a suggested canon of video works that is totally open to debate, open to updating and revising. The potential value of video art in medicine has been stressed along with pointers as to how these works might be used in specific clinical situations and in health education. As we've seen there are several important distinctions between video and standard cinematic productions. With video art it is much easier to be exposed for short periods and have multiple viewings. Ease of access via TikTok/YouTube/Vimeo and artists' own websites has been noted and the reference section below has many specific pointers to further works.

The distinction between cinema and video, between film as art and video as art, is porous. Unlike cinema – where, as outlined in Steven Schlozman's (2021) *Film*, there already exists a wealth of papers about its potential value in healthcare – video art has not, to any great extent as yet, been the subject of much scientific study as regards its potential impact on health and its use in clinical teaching. This book hopefully makes a case for further work in this area.

Academic study of video art and social platforms using video is still in its infancy. In 2005, a group at Amsterdam University of Applied Sciences set up the Institute of Network Cultures that in turn launched a project called Video Vortex in 2006. Since then this forum has become a lively research network organizing many European conferences and three anthologies of papers (Lovink & Treske,

2020). Their most recent, in 2020, points out that the critical vocabulary for video is still in evolution. They stress that there is, as yet, no canonical text that 'defines the depth and spread of online video'.

In the latest volume of Video Vortex there is much discussion about the 50-year journey from the Sony Portapak to the impact of 4K smartphones and their enormous influence on visual culture. Video as *evidence* is discussed as with its use by healthcare workers to demonstrate the catastrophic effect of the coronavirus on both patients and staff. Video was a *crucial* form of connection during the pandemic using the likes of Zoom and Google Teams apps. But it's not all doom and gloom. Thomas Elsaesser, the renowned German film historian, is quoted from the first volume of Video Vortex essays in 2008 as saying:

> *I have found on YouTube ways of knowing and ways of being that are ludic and reflective, educational and participatory, empowering and humbling ....*

Video Vortex repeatedly point out that one of the key advantages to video as art form, as educational tool, is that it gives us stories of 'an *edited* daily life' (italics mine). This is a crucial point. We're back to Christian Marclay's *The Clock* again – our problem with time. The use of time is a recurring theme among the interviewees discussed in *Gen Z, Explained* (Katz, Ogilvie, Shaw, & Woodhead, 2021). They mention one undergraduate reporting that

> *she and her friends rarely go to lectures. They have calculated how long it takes for them to cycle to the lecture, attend the lecture, and then cycle back to the dorm, and have decided instead to stay in their dorm rooms and watch a recording of the lecture. They watch it at triple speed: this is not only to save time, but also to help them stay attentive.*

Given the pressures on universities to pack as much into curricula as possible the radical editing of TikTok offers educators a way of achieving a faster and much more comprehensive approach to learning.

Social media platforms such as Twitter/YouTube/Facebook have already been used to train medical staff and provide learning for patients (Ventola, 2014; Kotsenas, Arce, Aase, Timini, Young & Wald, 2018). Healthcare workers can be seen teaching users about certain conditions (Nied, 2020). Platforms have been used specifically with the young to improve communication with patients (Hausmann, Touloumtzis, White, Colbert, & Gooding, 2017). And an estimated 84 per cent of US teenagers aged 13–18 years use Internet/digital tools for their *own* health information (Deardorff, 2016). Digital forms of health education are here to stay with the newest phenomenon being TikTok ....

TikTok was founded in 2017 and the app has more than 1 billion downloads (Zhu, Xu, Zhang, Chen, & Evans, 2019). Users are said to spend an average of 52 minutes per day (Bruno, 2020), 90 per cent of which do so on a daily basis. Bruno analysed 100 videos to understand how professionals are using TikTok and looked at self-recordings, demonstrations, information and education. This paper concluded that professionals are using TikTok to develop messaging likely to resonate with the young. The use of distinctive usernames to notify that the account is health-related was noted.

As Samantha Floreani (2023) writes: 'Is there any platform that creates as much collective angst as TikTok?' She goes on: 'For some TikTok is just a silly video app. For others, it's a symbol of our most potent social and political fears'. We read that the FBI has called the app 'a national security threat' (Clarke, 2023), that US government officials have to delete it from their phones. Worries about privacy and harm are real – anything that, say, encourages an eating disorder or self-harm cannot be good. Improper data access and its use as a propaganda tool cannot be excluded but these caveats are relevant to *all* social media platforms – it's the fact that the app comes from China that worries the West. However, as Floreani and this book argue, there *is* the potential for social good with such technology and if TikTok were to go down or banned it's highly likely that it would be replaced by a similar Western app.

So where are we with video art as of 2023? How is it viewed, as Art Monthly puts it, 'in an age defined on the one hand by inattention and on the other by an unprecedented level of individual agency'? Mimi Howard's (2023) essay 'On Viewing Video' tells us: 'As video journalism, short-form documentaries, iPhone reportage and Zoom Classes became essential aspects of the media landscape, so too did digital video art bend itself towards a dissociative, didactic, forensic mode that dealt in providing proof and paper trails – or "evidence of damage"'. Howard cites Forensic Architecture here – a collective that is 'exceptionally good at supplying the viewer – sometimes a literal court of law – with overwhelming evidence about human rights abuses'. This is video art working as a means of protection, as a defender of health and health rights.

There's no doubt that art institutions in 2023 have, what Howard calls, a voracious appetite for site-specific investigative video works. Howard cites the most recent Whitney Biennial where 30 per cent of the total catalogued works were video-based. A few are 'sometimes unstructured ... and sometimes something like academic research by other means'. There's an obvious overlap with the educational sector. Some may, Howard admits, 'have a grating and depressing effect on the audience'. This has to be admitted. There may be 'too much evidence of damage and not enough pathways to overcoming it', a not uncommon occurrence in contemporary medical practice.

There's also the concern mentioned earlier that there is a 'cognitive burden of digesting only so much information in so little time'. And this too, that the artwork 'sometimes morally implies the due diligence of watching a video all the way through'. The artist Alfredo Jaar acknowledges what Howard calls 'shrivelled-up attention-spans' and has capped one of his video works at five minutes with strict entry times. As Howard concludes, 'we remain in an experimentation phase in which the most appropriate way to show collected video work is yet to be discovered'. We are living through the 'growing pains of a genre'.

Contra the Situationist thinking of Guy Debord and that of critic T. J. Clark who worry that video and TV may be understood as a mere dehumanizing 'spectacle', I'd argue that it is not *all* bad. Not all of it screams 'get out of my mind' *a la* David Bowie. We need to be more selective in our approach to the medium, more open, and less frightened of its risks. Returning to the fluvial metaphor of my introduction we need to hold on to some of the solid rocks dotting our path without being shipwrecked and recognize which videos are a safe haven of truth. In many ways videos, the artworks and all those excerpts from TV on social media are like feuilletons, small articles in a magazine that we file away in our brains. We *are* equipped to do this, we can filter; our brains are better than we think they are. Media surfing can feel like we're on stormy seas, like we're white-water rafting, but it *can* be exhilarating, liberating. We may feel like we're drowning but actually we're waving. It's easy to blot out the materialistic demands to buy, buy, buy: just press the *skip ads* message and learn something ....

One of the standard traditional models of active clinical teaching in medical schools is ward-based education where students are taken to a patient who then tells them their history. Clinical signs can be easily demonstrated at the bedside. This form of teaching will always be relevant – there's no substitute for the real experience of seeing with your own eyes such signs as jaundice, cyanosis, anaemia and so on. There will always be a role for video demonstrations on grand rounds of new techniques too. But the digital age offers real advancements. YouTube/TikTok and other platforms can provide something entirely new to medicine. If you are teaching say, neurology or endocrinology you might have to wait months or *years* for a rare case to turn up on the ward or clinic. TikTok offers the incredible reality of witnessing ten cases of a rare condition, such as acromegaly or myotonia dystrophica mentioned earlier, in a mere 10 minutes.

One could make an argument for teaching the theory of a condition, its features and so on, in a lecture/seminar/symposium then breaking up for 15 minutes for students to explore the condition on several patient's own TikTok, Instagram or YouTube videos. The group could then reconvene to discuss these/quiz the lecturer further.

As discussed, there is an enormous archive of easy-to-access self-produced short videos by patients on TikTok, a fraction of which I've collected in the reference section. There will be other interesting examples I'm sure. I've argued there could be a place for institutional approval of some of these – a gold standard 'kite' mark if you like.

Compilations of such self-portrait videos by patients with ulcerative colitis or diabetes will never replace actual encounters with real patients but, in terms of time saved, I feel certain these will have a significant place in the medical education of the future if not already in the present. The age-old apprenticeship model on the wards will remain but we no longer have to wait decades to meet that patient with androgen insensitivity syndrome or phaeochromocytoma, encounter that individual coping with myasthenia gravis or cystic fibrosis.

I want to end my selection of videos by recommending a classic work that can act as a paradigm for medical education, indeed much of medical practice itself: Fischli and Weiss' *The Way Things Go* (1987). Like life itself, the film is funny and incessant, difficult and joyous. We see a seemingly endless chain of objects – 100 feet long in total – that includes tires, ladders, oil drums, water and soap. The work is about how each connects with one another as we watch a chain reaction of things pushing other things further and further along a seemingly never-ending journey to an unknown destination. Stuff burns and objects move down ramps, substances dissolve. What does this tell us? This artwork asks, quite plainly, that we must always consider the consequences of action: that momentum will out. This is as good a lesson for those involved in healthcare as any other. With all our knowledge, all our wisdom and experience, we should always remember that doing *this* might lead to *that*. That doing nothing is doing something too. That everything has consequences. Video is alert to this. We can be sure we'll be watching more and more in the future.

APPENDIX

VIDEO SOURCES

YouTube

Vito Acconci – Security Zone (1971)
Bas Jan Ader – Compilation of Works
Bas Jan Ader – Here Is Always Somewhere Else Documentary by Rene Daalder
Ed Atkins – Ribbons (2014)
Ed Atkins in conversation with Hans Ulrich Obrist (2015)
Mirosław Bałka – Fragment. Akadamie der Kunste, Berlin (2011)
Matthew Barney – The Cremaster Cycle
Meriem Bennani – Guided Tour of a Spill. Ghebaly (2021)
Dara Birnbaum – Technology/Transformation: Wonder Woman (1978–1979)
Christine Borland – Simbodies & Nobodies (2009)
Christine Borland – SimMan (2007), SimBaby (2008), SimWoman (2010)
Stan Brakhage – Autopsy: The Act of Seeing with One's Own Eyes (1971)
Candice Breitz – Love Story (2016)
Chris Burden – Shot in the Name of Art. New York Times
Chris Burden – The TV Commercials. MOCAtv
Vanessa Daws – At Home in the Water (2022) Fabrica Gallery
Wim Delvoye – Super Cloaca (2015)
Wim Delvoye – Louisiana Channel (2017)
Jacqueline Donachie – Inherited Characteristics
Tracey Emin – Why I Never Became a Dancer (1995)

Tracey Emin on Recovering from Cancer: Newsnight (2021)
Fischli and Weiss – The Way Things Go (1987)
Luke Fowler – All Divided Selves (2011) via Lux
Douglas Gordon – 10ms^{-1} (1994)
Douglas Gordon – Îles Flottantes
Douglas Gordon and Charles Esche in conversation BAK (2009)
Rebecca Horn, Berlin 1974
Robert Hughes - The Shock of the New
Arthur Jafa – Love Is the Message, The Message is Death (2016)
Arthur Jafa – Not All Good, Not All Bad. Louisiana Channel (2019)
Sin Wai Kin – Tate Shots (2022)
Katarzyna Kozyra – Men's Bathhouse (1999)
Erik Van Lieshout – Video on Maureen Paley Gallery Website (2022)
Paul McCarthy – 'All for the Gut' HENI Talks
Steve McQueen – Retrospective at Schaulager Basel (2013)
Christian Marclay – The Clock
Christian Marclay/On Time discussing The Clock
Bruce Nauman – Walking in an Exaggerated Manner Around the
Perimeter of a Square (1967–1968)
Bruce Nauman – At the Punta della Dogana, Venice
Yoko Ono – Cut Piece
Tony Oursler – Tunic (Song for Karen) (1990)
Adrian Piper – Cornered (1988)
Dennis Potter – Seeing the Blossom – the Last Interview (1994)
Pipilotti Rist – Ever Is Over All (1997)
Pipilotti Rist – Blutclip (1993)
Pipilotti Rist – Sip My Ocean (1996)
Martha Rosler – Semiotics of the Kitchen (1975)
Ryan Trecartin – I-Be Area (2007)
Ryan Trecartin – Junior War (2013)
Bill Viola – Nantes Triptych (1992)
Bill Viola – Louisiana Channel (2013)
Jenni-Juulia Wallinheimo-Heimonen – Battle of Scarcity of
Resources (2017)
Gillian Wearing – Wearing Masks (2012)
Jordan Wolfson – Raspberry Poseur (2012)

Jordan Wolfson – Real Violence (2017)
Lu Yang – Uterus Man (2013)

TikTok

@addiwithoutthee
@annaleahart
@careersdoctoruk
@hiddenstitchesuk
@shaniesfight
@winnieharlow

Twitter

@charliersmith1

Facebook

Christian Boltanski – L'homme qui tosse/The Man Who Coughs (1969) uploaded by kitchenartist
Ger van Elk: The Flattening of the Brooke's Surface (1972)

Vimeo

Christian Boltanski: Subliminal and Les Disparus
Christine Borland: Endless Walk (1999)
Katarzyna Kozyra – *Bathhouse* (1997)

Film

All the Beauty and the Bloodshed. Directed by Laura Poitras.

TV

My Dead Body: Channel 4

Recommended Websites Featuring Articles
and/or Videos on Video Art

Artform
Art Monthly
ArtReview
ArtForum
Guggenheim Museum
iMomus
Maureen Paley Gallery
Louisiana Channel
Vernissage TV
Goodman Gallery
Whitechapel Gallery

REFERENCES

Alaniz, M. H. (2022). Dangerous TikTok trends you should never try. Retrieved from Legacymarketing.com

Angermeyer, M. C., Matschinger, H., & Schomerus, G. (2013). Attitudes towards psychiatric treatment and people with mental illness: Changes over two decades. *British Journal of Psychiatry*, *203*(2), 146–151.

Bhasin, S., Brito, J. P., Cunningham, G. R., et al. (2018). Testosterone therapy in men with hypogonadism: An Endocrine Society clinical practice guideline. *Journal of Clinical Endocrinology and Metabolism*, *103*(5), 1715–1744.

Bradbury, N. A. (2016). Attention span during lectures: 8 seconds, 10 minutes, or more? *Advances in Physiological Education*, *40*, 509–513.

Bruno, C. M. (2020). A content analysis of how healthcare workers use TikTok. *Elon Journal of Undergraduate Research in Communications*, *11*(2), 5–16.

le Carré, J. (1979). *Smiley's people*. London: Hodder&Stoughton.

Clarke, L. (2023). TikTok: How the west has turned on Gen Z's favourite app. *Guardian*, February 5.

Colby, C. (2017). Steve McQueen's 'Ashes' haunts Institute of Contemporary Art. *Bay State Banner*, February 24.

Comp, G., Dyer, S., & Gottlieb, M. (2020). Is TikTok the next social media frontier for medicine? *AEM Education and Training*, *202*(1), 1–4.

Deardorff, J. (2016). Teens turn to Internet to cope with health challenges. Retrieved from northwestern.edu/stories/2015/06/teens-turn-to-internet-to-cope-with-health-challenges/

Donachie, J., & Monckton, D. G. (2006). *Tomorrow belongs to me.* Glasgow: University of Glasgow.

Donachie, J. (2016). *Illuminating loss: A study of the capacity for artistic practice to shape research and care in the field of inherited genetic disease.* Ph.D. thesis. Northumbria University.

Floreani, S. (2023). What are we worrying about when we worry about TikTok? *Guardian*, January 21.

Geniole, S. N., Bird, B. M., McVittie, J. S., Purcell, R. B., Archer, J. M., & Carré, J. M. (2020). Is testosterone linked to human aggression? A meta-analytic examination of the relationship between baseline, dynamic, and manipulated testosterone on human aggression. *Hormones and Behaviour, 123,* 104644.

Godfrey, M., Obrist, H. U., & Gillick, L. (2006). *Anri Sala.* London: Phaidon Press.

Goffman, E. (1963). *Stigma: Notes on the management of spoiled identity.* Penguin Modern Classics. Eaglewood cliffs, NJ: Prentice-Hall Inc.

Gordon, D. (2006). *Superhumanatural.* Edinburgh: National Gallery of Scotland.

Grinspoon, P. (2022). *The health effects of too much gaming.* Cambridge, MA: Harvard Health Publishing.

Hausmann, J. S., Touloumtzis, C., White, M. T., Colbert, J. A., & Gooding, H. C. (2017). Adolescent and young adult use of social media for health and its implications. *Journal of Adolescent Health, 60*(6), 714–719.

Howard, M. (2023). On viewing video. *Art Monthly, 463,* 6–10.

Jeffries, S. (2018). Jordan Wolfson: 'This is real abuse – not a simulation'. *Guardian*, May 3.

Katz, R., Ogilvie, S., Shaw, J., & Woodhead, L. (2021). *Gen Z, explained.* Chicago, IL: The University of Chicago Press.

Keefe, P. R. (2021). *Empire of pain.* New York, NY: Doubleday.

Knaak S., Mantler E., & Szeto A. (2017). *Mental-illness related stigma in healthcare: Barriers to access and care and evidence-based solutions* (pp. 111–116). Healthcare Management Forum. Los Angeles, CA: SAGE Publications.

Kotsenas, A. L., Arce, M., Aase, L., Timimi, F. K., Young, C., & Wald, J. T. (2018). The strategic imperative for the use of social media in healthcare. *Journal of the American College of Radiology, 15*(1), 155–161.

Kristeva, J. (1982). *The powers of horror: An essay on abjection.* New York, NY: Columbia University Press.

Kron, C. (2021). Artist Meriem Bennani's year of cultural vertigo. *Art Review*, May 7.

Laing, R. D. (1960). *The divided self.* Penguin Modern Classics.

Lifton R. J. (1986). *The Nazi doctors.* New York, NY: Basic Books.

London, B. (2020). *Video/art: The first fifty years.* London: Phaidon Press.

Lovink, G., & Treske, A. (Eds.). (2020). *Video Vortex Reader 3: Inside the YouTube decade.* Amsterdam: Institute of Network Cultures.

Debbaut J., Gordon, D., & McKee, F.1998). *Douglas Gordon: Kidnapping.* Eindhoven: Art Data.

Mangan, L. (2022). My dead body review – The skull crack makes even the medical students wince. *Guardian*, December 5.

Mitchell C., de Lange N., & Molestsane R. (2017). *Participatory visual methodologies: Social change, community and policy.* Thousand Oaks, CA: Sage.

Moran, J. (2023). Gen Z and me. *London Review of Books, 45*(4), 20–21.

Nabhan, Z. M., & Eugster, E. A. (2019). Testotoxicosis with an episodic course: An unusual case within a series. *AACE Clinical Case Reports, 5*(1), e50–e53.

Nabokov, V. (1951). *Speak, memory: An autobiography revisited.* London: Victor Gollancz..

Nabokov, V. (1955). 'On a book entitled *Lolita*', Afterword to *Lolita.* New York, NY: Putnam.

Nicolson, A. (2021). *Life between the tides.* London: William Collins.

Nied, J. (2020). Doctors are taking over TikTok to dish out important health information. Retrieved from www.shape.com/lifestyle/mind-and-body/doctors-on-tiktok

O'Doherty, B. (1976). *Inside the white cube: The ideology of the gallery space*. Oakland, CA: University of California Press.

O'Hagan, S. (2014). Nan Goldin: 'I wanted to get high from a really early age'. *Observer*, March 23.

Paik, N. J. to Porter McCray, 17/2/71. JDR 3rd Fund program files as cited in *Video Art* by Barbara London.

Pescosolido, B. A., Martin, J. K., Long, J. S., Medina, T. R., Phelan, J. C., & Link, B. G. (2010). "A disease like any other?" A decade of change in public relations to schizophrenia, depression, and alcohol dependence. *American Journal of Psychiatry*, *167*(11), 1321–1330.

Phelan, P., Obrist, H. U., & Bronfen, E. (2001). *Pipilotti Rist*. London: Phaidon Press.

Przybylski, A. K., Weinstein, N., & Murayama, K. (2017). Internet gaming disorder: Investigating the clinical relevance of a new phenomenon. *American Journal of Psychiatry*, *174*(3), 230–236.

Power 100: *Art Review* December 2021.

Royal College of Physicians. (2021). Social media principles and code of conduct. https://www.rcplondon.ac.uk/file/34951/download

Rugoff, R., Stiles, K., & Gioni, M. (2016). *Paul McCarthy*. London: Phaidon Press.

Sacks, O. (1984). *A leg to stand on*. London: Picador.

Sarkar, A. R. (2022). TikTok's 'blackout' challenge linked to deaths of 20 children in 18 months, report says. *Independent*, December 1.

Schlozman, S. (2021). *Film*. Bingley: Emerald Publishing.

Schwartz, A. (2017). Confronting the 'shocking' virtual reality work at the Whitney Biennial. *New Yorker*, March 20.

Semin, D., Garb, T., & Kupsit, D. B. (1997). *Christian Boltanski*. London: Phaidon Press.

Shen, G., Horikawa, T., Majima, K., & Kamitani, Y. (2019). Deep image reconstruction from human brain activity. *PLoS Computational Biology*, *15*(1), e1006633.

Stip, E., Caron, J., & Lane, C. J. (2001). Schizophrenia: People's perceptions in Quebec. *Canadian Medical Association Journal, 164*(9), 1299–1300.

Stone, J., Hewett, R., & Sharpe, M. (2008). The 'disappearance' of hysteria: Historical mystery or illusion? *Journal of the Royal Society of Medicine, 101*(1), 12–18.

Stone, J., Perthen, J., & Carson, A. J. (2012). 'A Leg to Stand On' by Oliver Sacks: A unique autobiographical account of functional paralysis. *Journal of Neurology, Neurosurgery and Psychiatry, 83*, 864–867.

Stuart, H., Chen, S. P., Christie, R., et al. (2014). Opening minds in Canada: Targeting change. *Canadian Journal of Psychiatry, 59*(10), S13–8.

Tomkins, C. (2014). Experimental people. The exuberant world of a video-art visionary. *New Yorker*, March 17.

Ventola, C. L. (2014). Social media and health care professionals: Benefits, risks, and best practices. *P&T: A Peer-reviewed Journal for Formulary Management, 39*(7), 491–520.

Walters, J. (2018). I don't know how they live with themselves – Artist Nan Goldin takes on the billionaire family behind Oxycontin. *Guardian*, January 22.

Wang, L., Zhou, L., Yang, W., & Yu, R. (2022). Deepfakes: A new threat to image fabrication in scientific publications? *Patterns, 3*(5), 100509.

Whitley, R., Sitter, K. C., Adamson, G., & Carmichael, V. (2020). Can participatory video reduce mental health stigma? Results from a Canadian action-research study of feasibility and impact. *BMC Psychiatry, 20*, article 16.

Wolfson, J. (2013). *Ecce Homo/le Poseur* (A. Moshayedi, Ed.), Köln: Walther König.

Zhu, C., Xu, X., Zhang, W., Chen, J., & Evans, R. (2019). How health communication via TikTok makes a difference: A content analysis of TikTok accounts run by Chinese provincial health committees. *International Journal of Environmental Research and Public Health, 17*(1), 192.

INDEX